Visual Guide for Clinicians

MULTIPLE SCLEROSIS

Ruth Dobson, MBBS, MA, MRCP
Clinical Research Fellow, Neuroimmunology Group
Blizard Institute, Barts and the London School of Medicine and Dentistry,
Queen Mary University of London, UK

and

Honorary SpR Neurology
Royal London Hospital, Barts Health NHS Trust
Whitechapel, London UK

Gavin Giovannoni, MBBCh, PhD, FCP(Neurol), FRCP, FRCPath
Professor of Neurology,
Blizard Institute, Barts and the London School of Medicine and Dentistry,
Queen Mary University of London, UK

and

Professor of Neurology
Royal London Hospital, Barts Health NHS Trust
London, UK

CLINICAL PUBLISHING
OXFORD

Clinical Publishing
an imprint of Atlas Medical Publishing Ltd
10 Innovation House, Parkway Court
Oxford Business Park South, Oxford OX4 2JY, UK

Tel: +44 1865 811116
Fax: +44 1865 251550
E mail: info@clinicalpublishing.co.uk
Web: www.clinicalpublishing.co.uk

Distributed in USA and Canada by:
Clinical Publishing
30 Amberwood Parkway
Ashland OH 44805, USA

Tel: 800-247-6553 (toll free within US and Canada)
Fax: 419-281-6883
Email: order@bookmasters.com

Distributed in UK and Rest of World by:
Marston Book Services Ltd
PO Box 269
Abingdon
Oxon OX14 4YN, UK

Tel: +44 1235 465500
Fax: +44 1235 465555
Email: trade.orders@marston.co.uk

© Atlas Medical Publishing Ltd 2013

First published 2013

All rights reserved. No part of this publication may be reproduced, stored in a retrieval system, or transmitted, in any form or by any means, without the prior permission in writing of Clinical Publishing or Atlas Medical Publishing Ltd

Although every effort has been made to ensure that all owners of copyright material have been acknowledged in this publication, we would be glad to acknowledge in subsequent reprints or editions any omissions brought to our attention

Clinical Publishing and Atlas Medical Publishing Ltd bear no responsibility for the persistence or accuracy of URLs for external or third-party internet websites referred to in this publication, and do not guarantee that any content on such websites is, or will remain, accurate or appropriate.

A catalogue record for this book is available from the British Library

ISBN-13   978 1 84692 096 7
e-ISBN   978 1 84692 639 6

The publisher makes no representation, express or implied, that the dosages in this book are correct. Readers must therefore always check the product information and clinical procedures with the most up-to-date published product information and data sheets provided by the manufacturers and the most recent codes of conduct and safety regulations. The authors and the publisher do not accept any liability for any errors in the text or for the misuse or misapplication of material in this work

Project manager: Gavin Smith, GPS Publishing Solutions, Herts, UK
Typeset by Phoenix Photosetting, Chatham, Kent, UK
Printed and bound by Marston Book Services Ltd, Abingdon, Oxon, UK

Contents

Contributors & Abbreviations	iv
1. Diagnosing multiple sclerosis *R Dobson, A Davis, B Turner*	1
2. Epidemiology of multiple sclerosis *A Handel, S Ramagopalan*	9
3. Magnetic resonance imaging in multiple sclerosis *K Schmierer*	17
4. Neurophysiology of multiple sclerosis *M Baker, C Blomberg*	23
5. Multiple sclerosis differential diagnosis and mimics *G Elrington*	31
6. Pathology of multiple sclerosis Part 1 – Human: *S Amor, P van der Valk* Part 2 – Animal models: *D Baker, S Al-Izki, K Lidster*	39
7. Treatment issues in multiple sclerosis *M Marta, M Papachatzaki*	51
8. Clinical outcome measures in multiple sclerosis *R Dobson, B Turner*	65
9. Neurorehabilitation in multiple sclerosis *A Neligan, J Buttell, C Liu*	71
Index	75

Contributors

Dr Sarah Al-Izki
Blizard Institute, Barts and the London School of Medicine and Dentistry, Queen Mary University of London, UK

Professor Sandra Amor
Department of Pathology, VU University Medical Center, Amsterdam, The Netherlands

Professor David Baker
Blizard Institute, Barts and the London School of Medicine and Dentistry, Queen Mary University of London, UK

Dr Mark Baker
Blizard Institute, Barts and the London School of Medicine and Dentistry, Queen Mary University of London, UK

Dr Cecilia Blomberg
Royal London Hospital, Barts Health NHS Trust, London, UK

Mr Joe Buttell
Regional Neurological Rehabilitation Unit, Homerton Hospital, London, UK

Dr Angharad Davis
Royal London Hospital, Barts Health NHS Trust, London, UK

Dr Giles Elrington
National Migraine Centre, London UK

Dr Adam Handel
Blizard Institute, Barts and the London School of Medicine and Dentistry, Queen Mary University of London, UK

Dr Katie Lidster
Blizard Institute, Barts and the London School of Medicine and Dentistry, Queen Mary University of London, UK

Dr Clarence Liu
Regional Neurological Rehabilitation Unit, Homerton Hospital, London, UK

Dr Monica Marta
Blizard Institute, Barts and the London School of Medicine and Dentistry, Queen Mary University of London, UK

Dr Aidan Neligan
National Hospital for Neurology and Neurosurgery, Queen Square, London, UK

Dr Maria Papachatzaki
Blizard Institute, Barts and the London School of Medicine and Dentistry, Queen Mary University of London, UK

Dr Sreeram Ramagopalan
Blizard Institute, Barts and the London School of Medicine and Dentistry, Queen Mary University of London, UK

Dr Klaus Schmierer
Blizard Institute, Barts and the London School of Medicine and Dentistry, Queen Mary University of London, UK

Dr Ben Turner
Royal London Hospital, Barts Health NHS Trust, London, UK

Professor Paul van der Valk
Department of Pathology, VU University Medical Center, Amsterdam, The Netherlands

Abbreviations

ADEM	acute disseminated encephalomyelitis
BBB	blood–brain barrier
CMCT	central motor conduction time
DMD	disease-modifying drug
DWI	diffusion-weighted image
EAE	experimental autoimmune encephalomyelitis
EBV	Epstein-Barr virus
EDSS	Expanded Disability Status Score
FAMS	Functional Assessment in MS
FLAIR	fluid attenuated inversion recovery
GA	glatiramer acetate
Gd+	gadolinium enhancing
HLA	human leucocyte antigen
IFN	interferon
IM	infectious mononucleosis
IV	inverse variance
JCV	JC (after John Cunningham) virus
LVEF	left ventricular ejection function
MS	multiple sclerosis
MSCF	Multiple Sclerosis Functional Composite
MSIS-29	MS Impact Scale 29
MSQL-54	MS Quality of Life-54
MUGA	multiple gated acquisition scan
MUS	medically unexplained symptoms
Nab	neutralizing antibody
OCB	oligoclonal band
ON	optic neuritis
PML	progressive multifocal leukoencephalopathy
PPMS	primary progressive multiple sclerosis
RF	radio-frequency
RNFL	retinal nerve fibre layer
RRMS	relapsing–remitting multiple sclerosis
S1P	sphingosine-1-phosphate
SPMS	secondary progressive multiple sclerosis
SSEP	somatosensory evoked potential
T	Tesla
VEP	visual evoked potential
WBC	white blood cell

Chapter 1
Diagnosing multiple sclerosis

Ruth Dobson, Angharad Davis and Ben Turner

Multiple sclerosis (MS) is an inflammatory disorder of the central nervous system (CNS) and the most common non-traumatic cause of neurodisability in the young.[1] The average age at diagnosis is approximately 30 years. Up to 50% of people with MS become unemployed within 8–10 years of diagnosis, highlighting the high personal and societal cost of this disorder.

Clinical presentation of MS

MS can present with a variety of clinical syndromes (*Table 1.1*). However, the disease almost always follows one of a few stereotyped courses (**1.1**), with associated paraclinical findings. Consensus criteria are available for the diagnosis of MS (*Table 1.2*). A number of 'red flags' prompt the physician to consider an alternative diagnosis (*Table 1.3*).

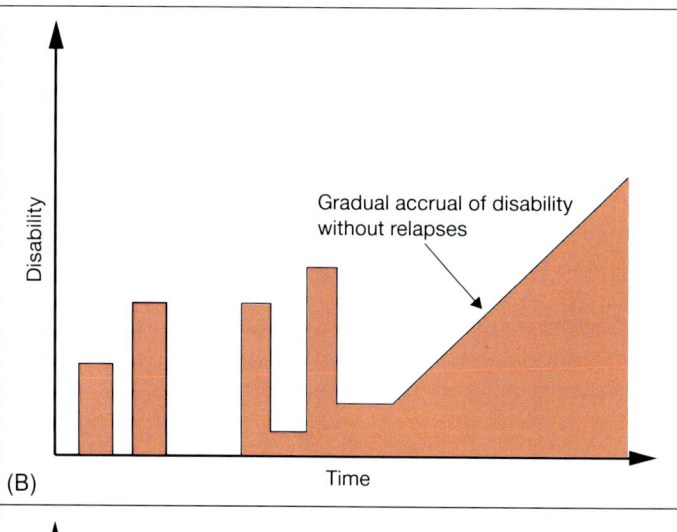

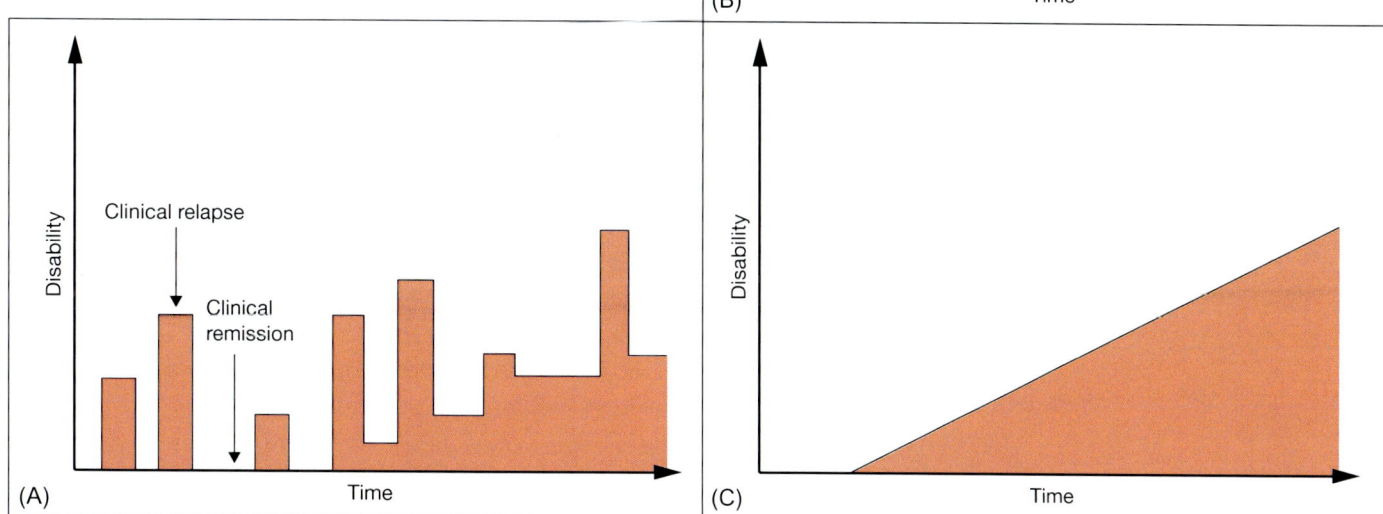

1.1 Subtypes of multiple sclerosis. (A) Relapsing–remitting MS is characterized by episodic neurological symptoms (relapses), lasting days to weeks, followed by complete or partial recovery. (B) Following relapsing–remitting MS, many patients go on to develop secondary progressive MS, with gradual accrual of disability independent of relapses. (C) Primary progressive MS is characterized by the absence of relapses and the gradual accrual of disability from disease onset.

Diagnosing multiple sclerosis

Table 1.1 Presenting symptoms in MS

Symptom/sign	Frequency (%)
Long tract symptoms (i.e. those arising from brain or spinal cord)	52
Multifocal symptoms	21
Optic neuritis	18
Brainstem symptoms	9

Adapted from Confavreux et al.[5]

Table 1.3 'Red flags' indicating that an alternative diagnosis to MS should be sought

- Age >60 years
- Hyperacute onset suggestive of vascular aetiology
- Lower motor neuron features, amyotrophy
- Significant nerve root pain
- MRI not in keeping with MS
- Features suggestive of an alternative multisystem disorder involving the CNS, such as aphthous ulcers, photosensitive rash

Table 1.2 McDonald criteria for the diagnosis of MS (2010)[6]

Clinical presentation	Additional data needed for MS diagnosis	
• ≥2 attacks AND objective clinical evidence of ≥2 lesions; OR • Objective clinical evidence of 1 lesion AND reliable history of ≥1 previous attack	None	
• ≥2 attacks AND objective clinical evidence of 1 lesion	Dissemination in space	• ≥1 T2 lesion in at least 2 of 4 'MS-typical' regions of the CNS (periventricular, juxtacortical, infratentorial or spinal cord); **OR** • Await a further clinical attack implicating a different site
• 1 attack AND objective clinical evidence of ≥2 lesions	Dissemination in time	• Simultaneous presence of gadolinium-enhancing and non-enhancing lesions on a single scan; **OR** • A new T2 and/or new gadolinium-enhancing lesion on a follow-up MRI; **OR** • Await a second clinical attack
• 1 attack AND objective clinical evidence of 1 lesion (clinically isolated syndrome)	Dissemination in time and space	• Dissemination in **time**: simultaneous presence of gadolinium-enhancing and non-enhancing lesions on a single scan, or a new T2 and/or new gadolinium-enhancing lesion on a follow-up MRI; **AND** • Dissemination in **space**: ≥1 T2 lesion in at least 2 of 4 'MS-typical' regions of the CNS (periventricular, juxtacortical, infratentorial or spinal cord); **OR** • Await a second clinical attack implicating a different site
• Insidious neurological progression suggestive of MS (primary progressive MS)	1 year of disease progression (prospective or retrospective)	• Evidence of dissemination in space on MRI of brain and/or spinal cord • Positive CSF oligoclonal bands and/or elevated IgG index

CNS, central nervous system; CSF, cerebrospinal fluid; IgG, immunoglobulin G; MRI, magnetic resonance imaging; MS, multiple sclerosis.

Approximately 85% of people with MS present with a relapse, defined as acute deterioration in neurological function, followed by partial or total recovery (remission). The symptoms experienced during a relapse are dependent on the site of the lesions, although certain presentations are more common (*Table 1.1*). The first clinical event is described as a clinically isolated syndrome.

If a patient has a second relapse or shows magnetic resonance imaging (MRI) evidence of active disease then they fulfil the criteria for clinically definite relapsing–remitting MS (RRMS). The probability of progression from clinically isolated syndrome to clinically definite MS is highly dependent on MRI and cerebrospinal fluid (CSF) findings.[2] Patients may have relapses for a number of years, and may accrue fixed disability with each relapse.

After disease duration of 10–25 years, patients with RRMS may begin to accrue disability independent of relapses. They are then described as having secondary progressive MS (SPMS). Patients with SPMS may or may not continue to have relapses.

A significant minority of patients (10–15%) present with a progressive course from the outset without relapses. These patients are described as having primary progressive MS (PPMS). Rarely, a patient with a PPMS course has superimposed relapses and this is then referred to as progressive relapsing MS.

If a patient has been diagnosed with MS for 15 years and remains independently mobile, then they are referred to as having 'benign MS'. This diagnosis can only be made in retrospect.

Common clinical presentations

Although patients with MS may present with any number of neurological deficits, there are a few clinical presentations that are particularly common and worthy of further discussion.

Optic neuritis
Approximately 20% of patients who go on to develop MS present with optic neuritis (ON). Not all patients with ON go on to develop MS, but the overwhelming majority of patients with MS have at least one episode of ON.

The diagnosis of ON is predominantly a clinical one. Patients complain of unilateral visual blurring and/or colour desaturation. This is typically associated with retro-orbital eye pain, which is exacerbated by eye movements. Symptoms develop over days, and an ongoing deterioration in vision after 2 weeks suggests an alternative diagnosis. In ON associated with MS, total visual loss is rare, and suggests an alternative underlying aetiology.

Examination of the fundus may reveal normal findings (**1.2**), or swelling of the disc, if the site of inflammation is anterior. The latter is referred to as papillitis and is seen in approximately 30% of patients presenting with ON (**1.3**). An afferent pupillary defect or relative afferent pupillary defect is commonly found, although this may be subtle in mild cases. Following resolution of an acute attack of ON, optic atrophy can be seen (**1.4**). MRI during an acute attack of ON may show gadolinium enhancement of the optic nerve sheath (**1.5**).

Treatment of an acute attack of ON is with intravenous steroids (most commonly methylprednisolone, 1 g/day for 3 days). This hastens recovery, but does not have any effect on long-term visual outcome.[3]

Transverse myelitis
There are a large number of causes of acute transverse myelitis, of which MS is only one. The clinical history tends to be that of evolution of weakness and/or sensory symptoms over days. Patients may have loss of pain, temperature and vibration sensation with a clear sensory level. Bladder and bowel function may also be affected.

Lhermitte's syndrome, in which neck flexion results in paraesthesia down the spine and in the upper and/or lower limbs has classically been associated with a demyelinating lesion in the cervical spinal cord. However, this sign is not pathognomonic of MS, and may be seen in other conditions such as compressive myelopathies. A rare manifestation

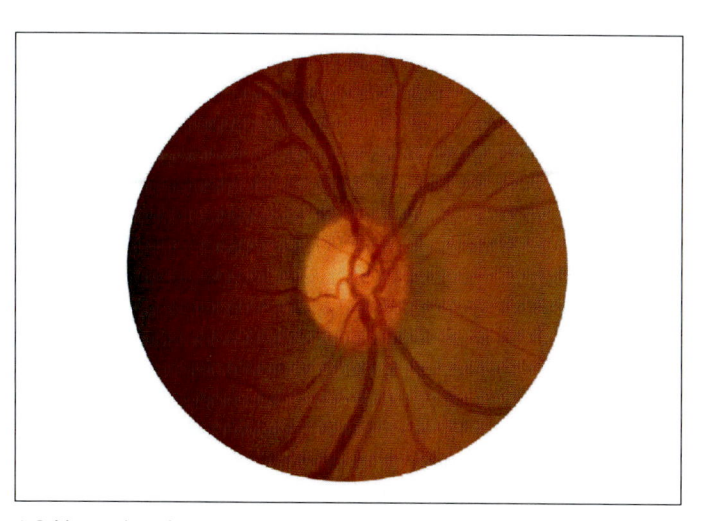

1.2 Normal optic disc.

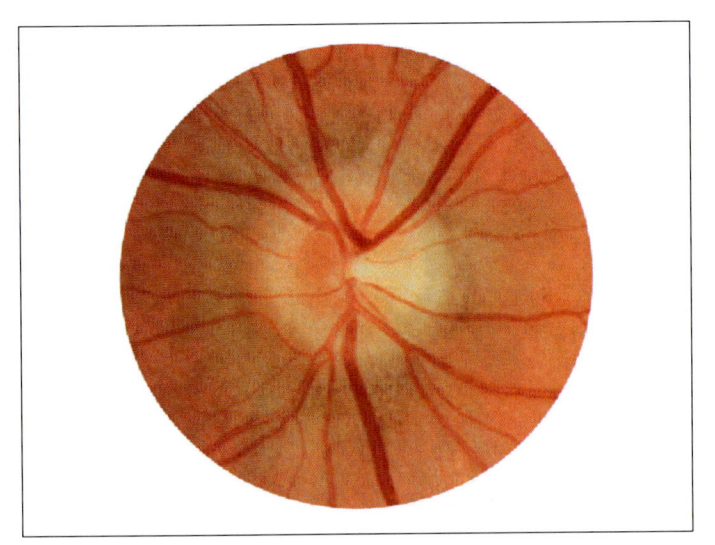

4 Diagnosing multiple sclerosis

1.3 Acutely inflamed disc (papillitis) in optic neuritis.

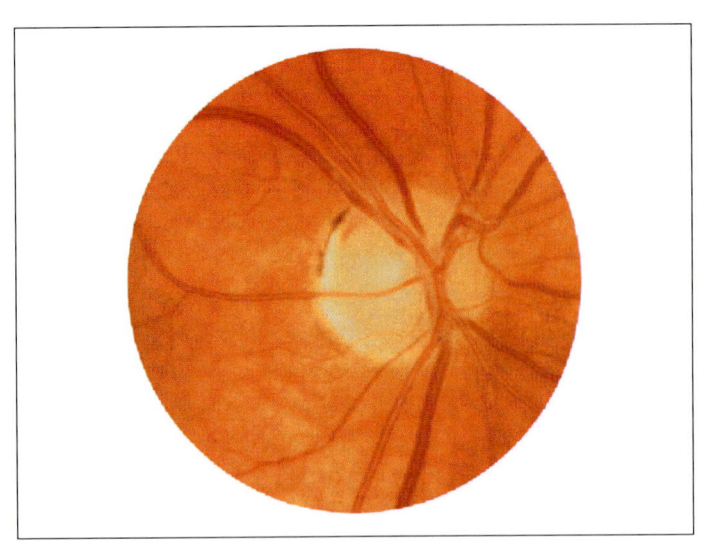

1.4 Optic atrophy.

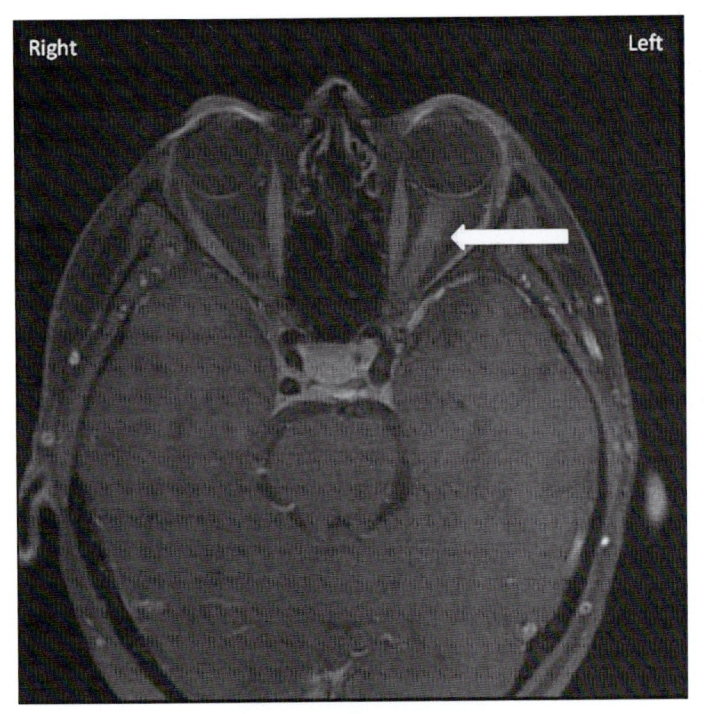

1.5 MRI showing gadolinium enhancement of the left optic nerve (*arrowed*) in keeping with acute optic neuritis.

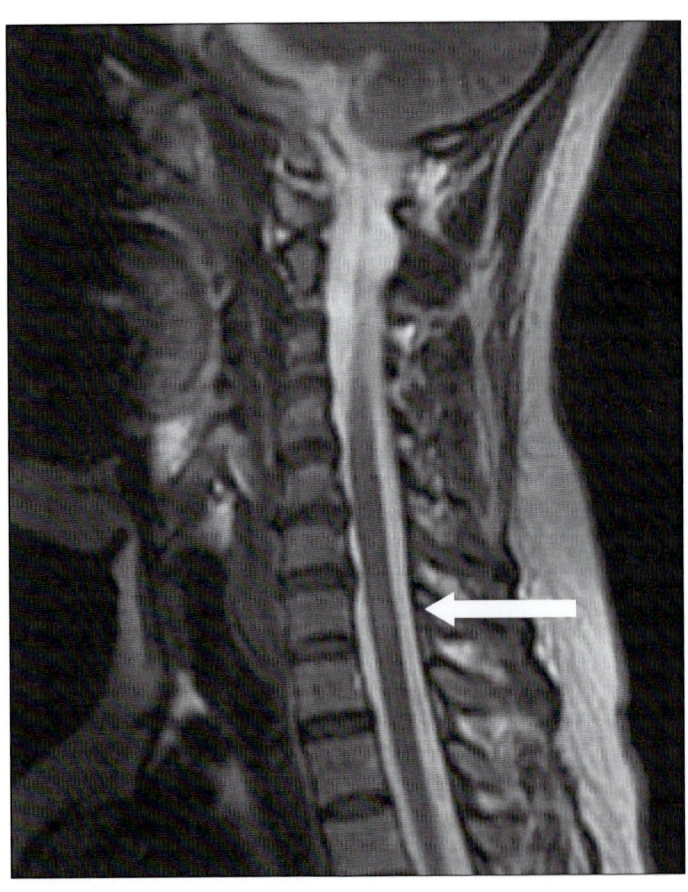

1.6 Typical image of a T2-hyperintense lesion within the spinal cord in keeping with transverse myelitis (*arrowed*).

is flexor spasms due to spontaneous activation of motor pathways. The spasms are usually self-limiting, resolve within 4–6 weeks, and they respond to sodium channel blockers (e.g. carbamazepine).

The diagnostic modality of choice for acute transverse myelitis is MRI. This may show a signal change within the spinal cord on T2-weighted sequences, with or without cord swelling (**1.6**). In MS, this signal change is typically asymmetric, and rarely exceeds two vertebral segments in length. Lesions longer than this are referred to as longitudinally extensive transverse myelitis and are more common in the MS mimic neuromyelitis optica (Devic's disease). In transverse myelitis associated with MS, lesions typical for MS may be seen elsewhere in the CNS.

Brainstem symptoms

Approximately 1 in 10 patients with MS will present with a brainstem syndrome. Common presentations include internuclear ophthalmoplegia, which can be bilateral (caused by bilateral lesions affecting the medical longitudinal fasciculi), ataxia with nystagmus, sixth nerve palsy and facial numbness.[4] Less commonly, facial palsy, trigeminal neuralgia, hemifacial spasm, facial myokymia and other ophthalmoplegias may be seen.

A number of brainstem syndromes are not commonly associated with MS. These include complex and complete external ophthalmoplegia, third nerve palsy, progressive trigeminal neuralgia and focal dystonia with or without torticollis. Multiple cranial neuropathies should prompt the search for an alternative diagnosis.[4]

Investigation findings

Blood tests

Routine blood tests are usually normal in MS. The role of blood tests is, therefore, predominantly in the elimination of other potential diagnoses, which are discussed in more detail in Chapter 5.

Cerebrospinal fluid

The majority of patients diagnosed with MS will have CSF analysis performed. Typical findings are described in *Table 1.4*. Although CSF analysis is only included in the diagnostic criteria for PPMS, it is often examined in cases where RRMS is suspected. CSF examination is important in suspected MS as it can both support the diagnosis of MS and exclude alternative diagnoses.

Table 1.4 Typical CSF findings in MS

- CSF may show mild pleocytosis (<50×10⁶ leucocytes/l), predominantly neutrophils
- Unmatched oligoclonal bands unique to cerebrospinal fluid
- Raised CSF IgG index indicating central nervous system production of IgG
- Protein typically normal or slightly raised
- Glucose typically normal

CSF samples are obtained via lumbar puncture (**1.7**). While this has traditionally been performed using cutting needles (otherwise known as traumatic or Quinke needles),

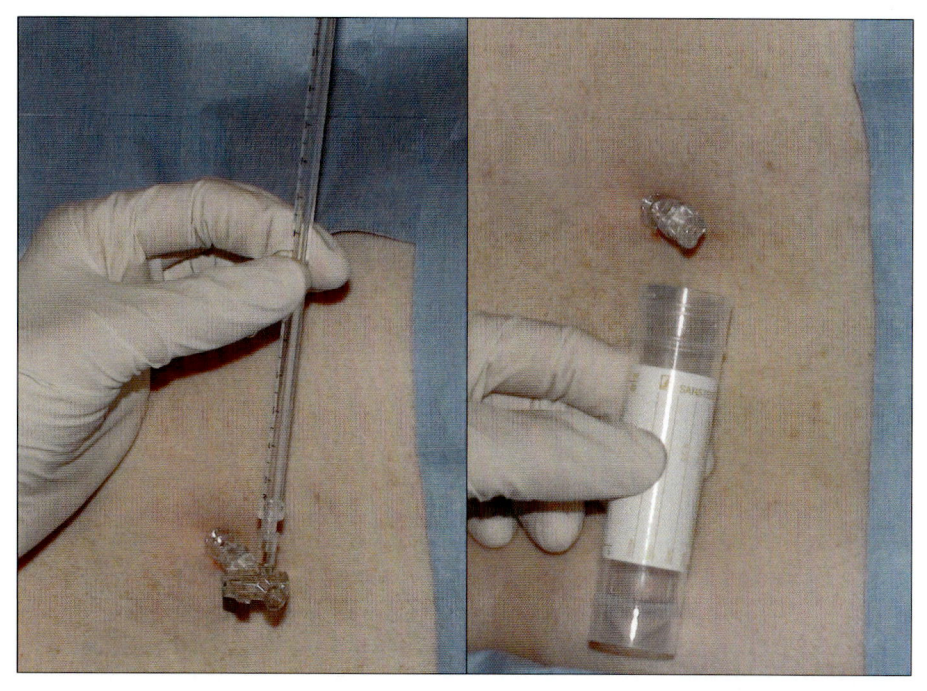

1.7 Performing a lumbar puncture. The patient is in the left lateral position, and the L3/4 interspace identified. The area is infiltrated with local anaesthetic and the spinal needle inserted. A manometer is used to measure CSF pressure before CSF collection. Reference 7 is a good online video on how to perform a lumbar puncture.

6 Diagnosing multiple sclerosis

there is a move towards the use of atraumatic needle systems (Sprotte) (**1.8**). These have been shown to reduce the rates of post-lumbar puncture headache in those undergoing diagnostic lumbar puncture.

CSF should be collected in a polypropylene tube (**1.9**). Basic CSF parameters (protein and glucose) are usually normal. Although there may be a slight elevation in the CSF white cell count, particularly in the context of an acute relapse, this tends not to be marked.

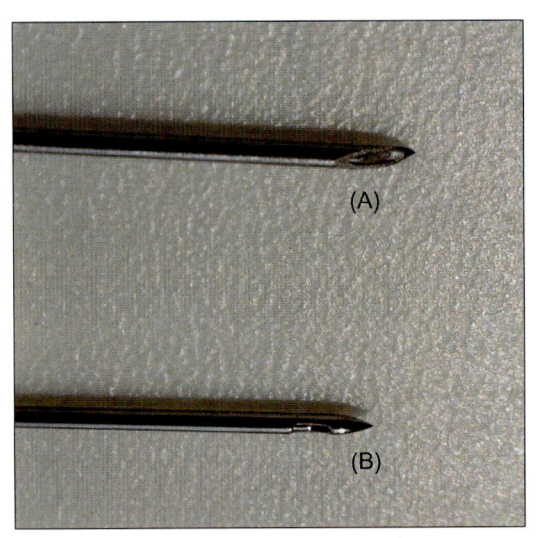

1.8 (A) Traumatic (Quincke) and (B) atraumatic (Sprotte) needle systems used in lumbar puncture. The 'pencil-point' tip of the atraumatic needle system can clearly be seen. This prevents the formation of a persistent dural flap with CSF leak, which is thought to be responsible for the occurrence of post-lumbar puncture headache.

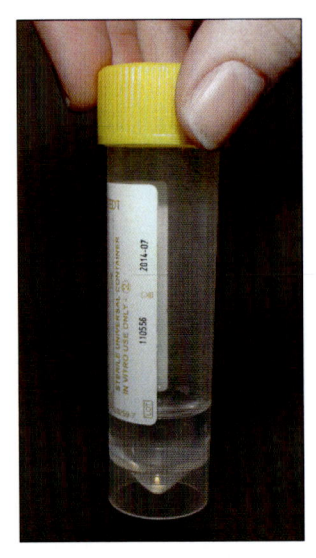

1.9 Clear and colourless CSF collected in a polypropylene tube.

The hallmark of MS is the presence of CSF oligoclonal IgG bands (**1.10**), which are present in more than 90% of patients. These represent the intrathecal synthesis of oligoclonal immunoglobulin G (IgG), which is unique to the CSF, and not present in a paired serum sample. Oligoclonal bands are detected using isoelectric focusing with immunofixation. It must be noted that oligoclonal bands are not specific for MS, as they may be present in a number of conditions, including CNS infections, CNS lupus and other autoimmune disease (e.g. paraneoplastic syndromes). Their presence is therefore merely supportive of a diagnosis of MS and should be interpreted alongside clinical history. The absence of oligoclonal bands is very useful in excluding a diagnosis of MS (i.e. their negative predictive value).

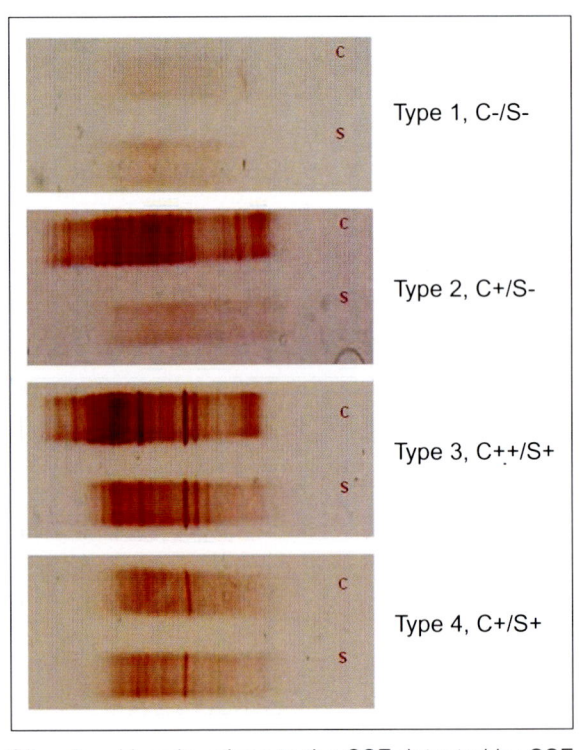

1.10 Oligoclonal bands unique to the CSF detected by CSF isoelectric focusing; the oligoclonal bands present are due to IgG. There are four common patterns: type 1, no bands in CSF and serum (S); type 2, oligoclonal IgG bands in CSF, not in the S sample, indicative of intrathecal IgG synthesis; type 3, oligoclonal bands in CSF (like type 2) and additional identical oligoclonal bands in CSF and the S sample – the unique CSF bands are indicative of intrathecal IgG synthesis; type 4, identical oligoclonal bands in CSF and the S sample illustrative of a systemic rather than intrathecal immune reaction, with a leaky or normal or abnormal blood–CSF barrier and oligoclonal bands passively transferred in the CSF.

Diagnosing multiple sclerosis

Magnetic resonance imaging

The typical MRI finding seen in MS is multifocal demyelination. This is visualized as T2-weighted hyperintensities seen on unenhanced MRI (**1.11**). Acute lesions may enhance after administration of gadolinium. The MRI findings in MS are discussed in more detail in Chapter 3.

Neurophysiology

The role of neurophysiology in the diagnosis of MS will be discussed more in Chapter 4. Suffice to say, the main value of neurophysiology is to show central conduction slowing, which is pathognomonic of demyelination. Conduction slowing is useful to show subclinical involvement of specific pathways, which often helps to show dissemination of lesions in space.

Differential diagnosis

An accurate diagnosis of MS is dependent on both the exclusion of plausible alternative diagnoses, the range of which may depend on presenting symptoms and signs, as well as a clinical picture in keeping with MS. The differential diagnosis of MS is covered in more detail in Chapter 5.

Online resources for patients and practitioners

Online resources can be a valuable source of information and support for both patients and practitioners. A number of websites are particularly recommended (*Table 1.5*).

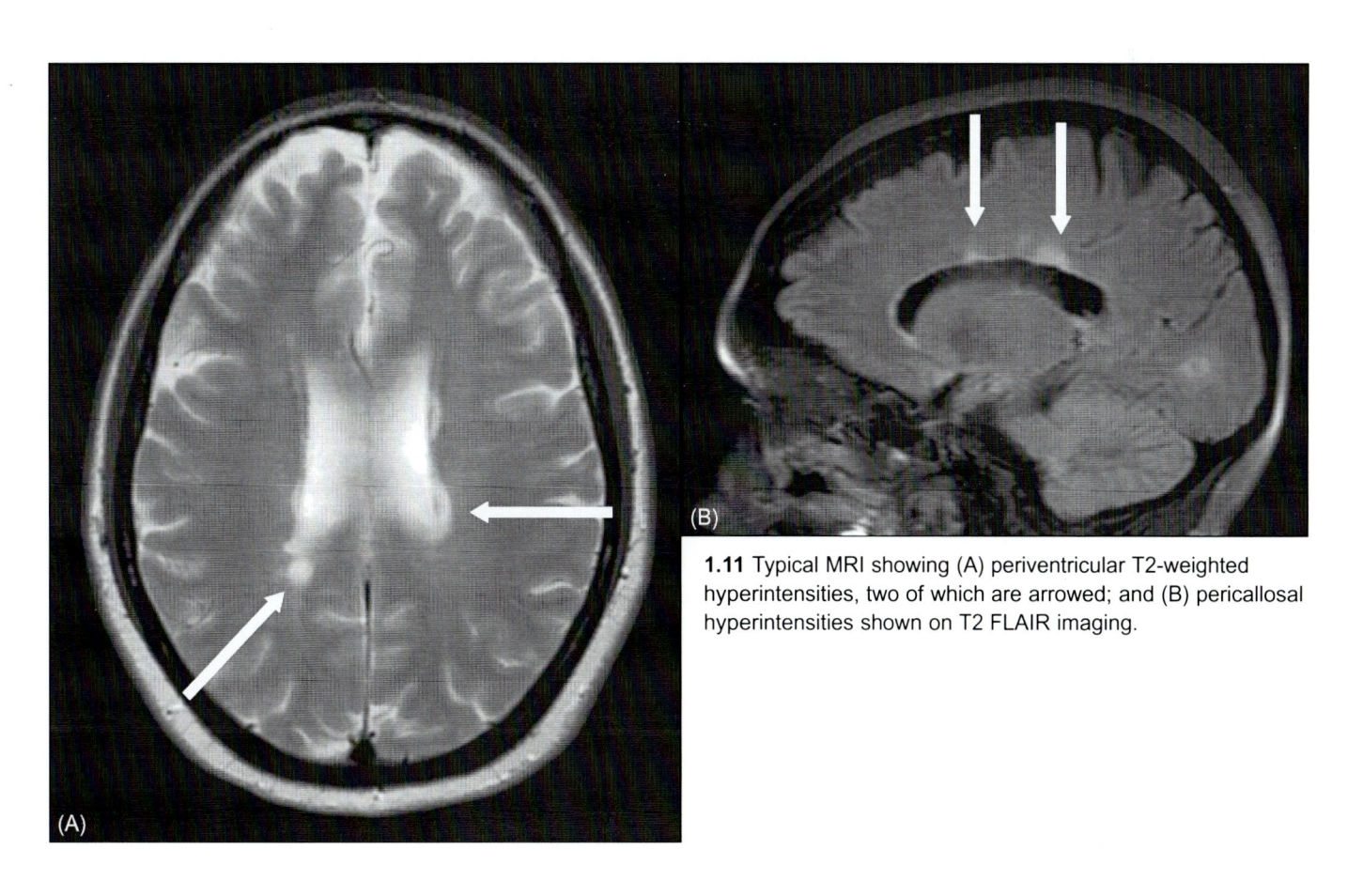

1.11 Typical MRI showing (A) periventricular T2-weighted hyperintensities, two of which are arrowed; and (B) pericallosal hyperintensities shown on T2 FLAIR imaging.

Table 1.5 Online resources for people with MS, and those with an interest in MS

Resource	Web address
MS Society of Great Britain and Northern Ireland	www.mssociety.org.uk/
MS Trust	www.mstrust.org.uk/
Shift MS – for young people with MS	http://shift.ms/
Multiple Sclerosis blog	www.multiple-sclerosis-research.blogspot.co.uk/
Multiple Sclerosis Resource Centre	www.msrc.co.uk/
National MS Therapy Centres	www.msntc.org.uk/
National MS Society (North America)	www.nationalmssociety.org
Multiple Sclerosis International Federation (MSIF)	www.msif.org/en/

References

1. Hauser S, Oksenberg J. The neurobiology of multiple sclerosis: genes, inflammation, and neurodegeneration. *Neuron* 2006; **52**: 61–76.
2. Tintore M, Rovira A, Rio J, *et al*. Do oligoclonal bands add information to MRI in first attacks of multiple sclerosis? *Neurology* 2008; **70**(13 Pt 2): 1079–83.
3. Beck RW, Cleary PA. Optic neuritis treatment trial. One-year follow-up results. *Arch Ophthalmol* 1993; **111**(6): 773–5.
4. Miller DH, Weinshenker BG, Filippi M, *et al*. Differential diagnosis of suspected multiple sclerosis: a consensus approach. *Multiple Sclerosis* 2008; **14**(9): 1157–74.
5. Confavreux C, Vukusic S, Moreau T, Adeleine P. Relapses and progression of disability in multiple sclerosis. *N Engl J Med* 2000; **343**(20): 1430–8.
6. Polman CH, Reingold SC, Banwell B, *et al*. Diagnostic criteria for multiple sclerosis: 2010 revisions to the McDonald criteria. *Ann Neurol* 2011; **69**(2): 292–302.
7. Ellenby MS, Tegtmeyer K, Lai S, Braner DAV. Lumbar puncture. [Video] *N Engl J Med* 2006; 355: e12. Available at www.youtube.com/watch?v=Z_TMizgIHPA. [Accessed 15 October 2012].

Chapter 2

Epidemiology of multiple sclerosis

Adam E. Handel and Sreeram V. Ramagopalan

Global distribution of MS

The prevalence of MS varies markedly throughout the world from <5/100 000 in some parts of Asia to >200/100 000 in the Orkney Islands (**2.1**).[1] There is a clear latitudinal gradient for disease prevalence whereby MS is more common further from the Equator.[2] This gradient can be observed within several countries suggesting that this latitudinal effect is likely to be mediated by environmental risk factors rather than solely by genetic differences between populations.[3–6]

Sex ratio

A key observation in MS epidemiology is the excess of female cases compared with male cases.[7] In most European populations this is a female-to-male ratio of approximately 2:1. However, there is evidence that the sex ratio has not always been as elevated as this and appears to have changed markedly over the last 100 years; a trend likely to be explained by altered exposure to environmental risk factors (**2.2**).[8,9] The sex ratio is not uniform for different subtypes of MS: PPMS, constituting approximately 20% of patients, has a sex ratio of approximately 1:1, whereas RRMS has a sex ratio of 2–3:1.[7] In paediatric or childhood-onset MS the sex ratio is also 1:1.

Migration studies in MS

Epidemiological studies of immigrants are particularly informative for suggesting windows of time in which environmental risk factors act to determine MS

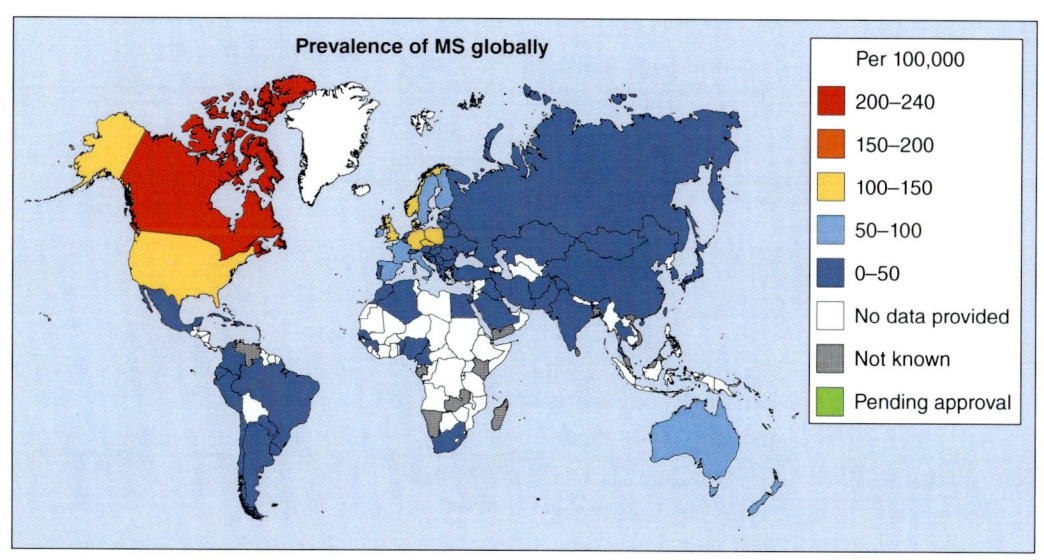

2.1 Global prevalence of multiple sclerosis. Data from the *Atlas of MS* showing prevalence per 100 000 population in 2008.[1]

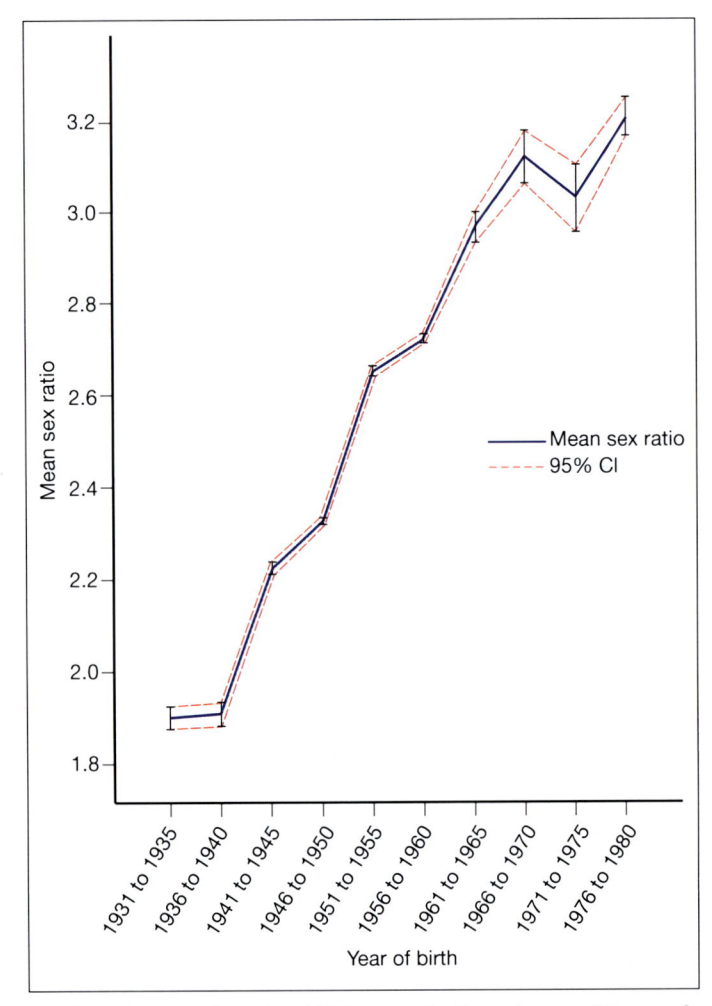

2.2 Female-to-male ratio of MS cases in Canada over 50 years.[8]

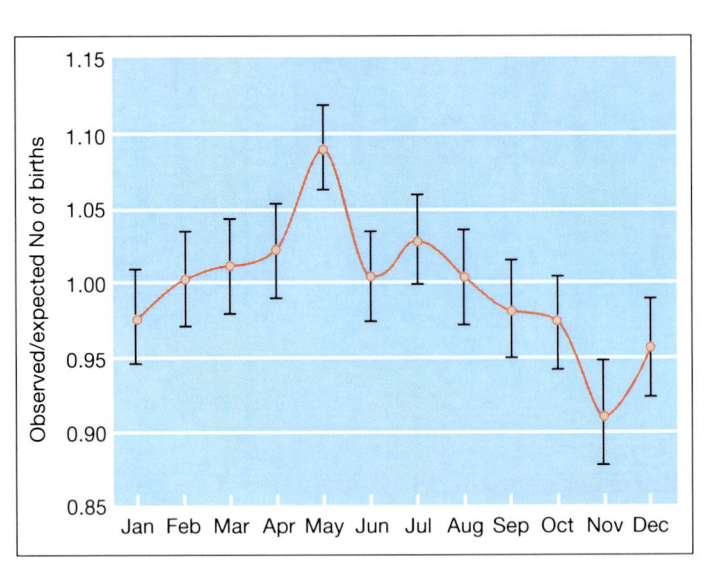

2.3 Month of birth effect in MS. Observed/expected number of births for a combined cohort of Canadian, British, Danish and Swedish births.[13]

susceptibility. Individuals older than approximately 15 years of age at the time of migration retain the MS risk of their country of origin and those younger than this have a risk close to natives.[10–12] This suggests that adolescence and early adulthood constitutes a window of time during which MS susceptibility is altered by environmental exposures.

Month of birth and MS

The risk of MS has been found to vary depending upon the month in which an individual is born. In the northern hemisphere, MS susceptibility is greatest for those born in May and lowest for those born in November (**2.3**).[13] Interestingly, this pattern is reversed in the southern hemisphere, strongly suggesting that a seasonal risk factor, presumably acting *in utero* modifies MS risk later in life.[14]

Genetics and MS susceptibility

Nearly 20% of patients with MS report another family member with MS.[15] It is therefore unsurprising that genetics is an important determinant of MS susceptibility. The risk of MS in relatives of patients with MS differs depending upon relationship (**2.4**).[16] However, MS genetic susceptibility is not simply the degree of relatedness, as a parent-of-origin effect occurs whereby maternal relations are at increased risk of MS compared with paternal relations (**2.5**).[17–19]

Until recently, the only firmly established genetic association was with the human leucocyte antigen (HLA) locus on chromosome 6, particularly with the haplotype

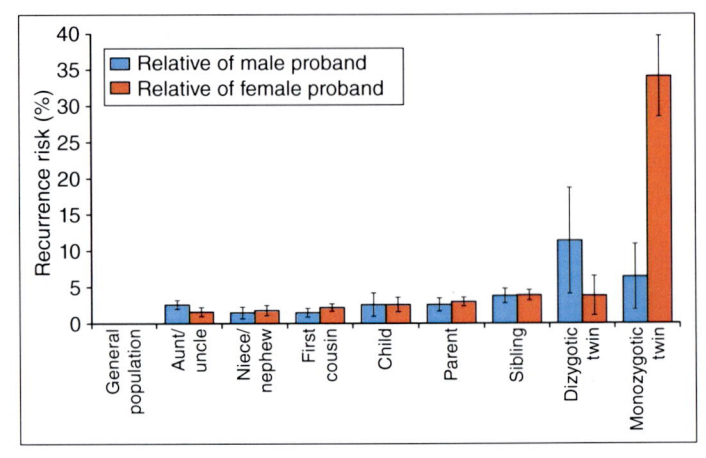

2.4 Familial recurrence risk in MS for differing degrees of relatedness.[16]

Epidemiology of multiple sclerosis

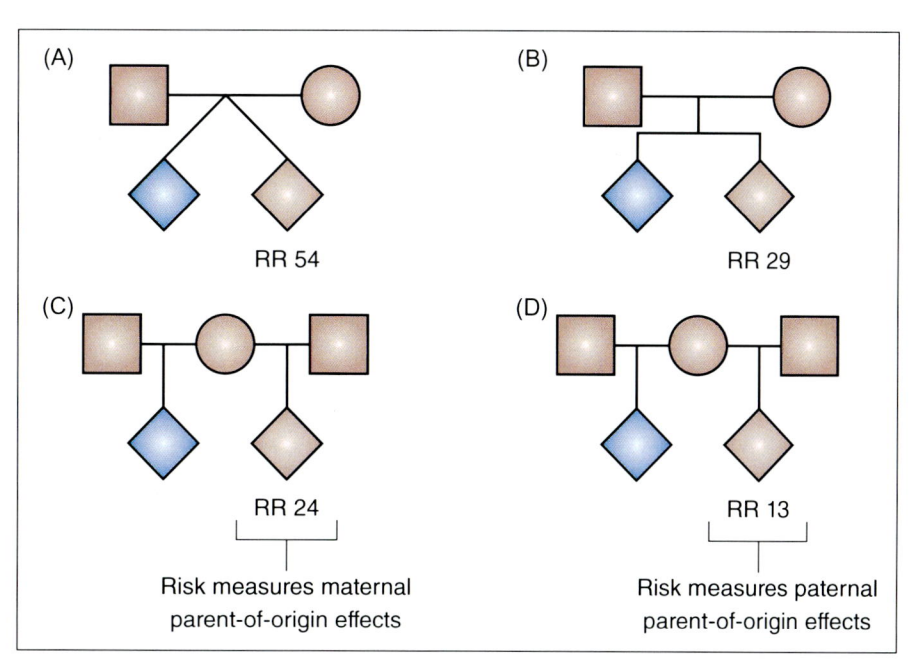

2.5 Pedigree diagram showing maternal parent-of-origin effects in MS. Age-corrected relative risk (RR) of recurrence for (A) dizygotic twins, (B) full siblings, (C) maternal half siblings and (D) paternal half siblings was calculated assuming a background prevalence of MS of 100 cases per 100 000 individuals. Squares represent males and circles represent females. Blue symbols represent individuals diagnosed as having MS.[26]

HLA-DRB1*1501-DQA*0102-DQB*0602.[20] The situation is more complicated than a single risk haplotype, however, as interactions between different alleles at *HLA-DRB1* determine MS genetic susceptibility at this locus (**2.6**).[21]

Since 2007 there has been a rapid proliferation in genome-wide association studies, leading to the identification of 57 common genetic variants outside of the *HLA* region associated with MS susceptibility.[22] These individually have modest odds ratios (1.08–1.26) but are an important component in determining overall genetic risk of MS. Most risk loci contain genes encoding immunological proteins, supporting the view that MS is primarily an autoimmune condition.

Identifying rare variants associated with MS susceptibility requires approaches using genetic sequencing methodologies. Whole exome sequencing (sequencing all protein coding genes) of families with a high frequency of MS and subsequent genotyping of large cohorts of patients and controls revealed rare variants in *CYP27B1*, a gene responsible for vitamin D1α-hydroxylation.[23] Vitamin D deficiency is an important risk factor for MS and so the identification of this rare variant provides a strong link between environmental and genetic determinants of MS susceptibility.

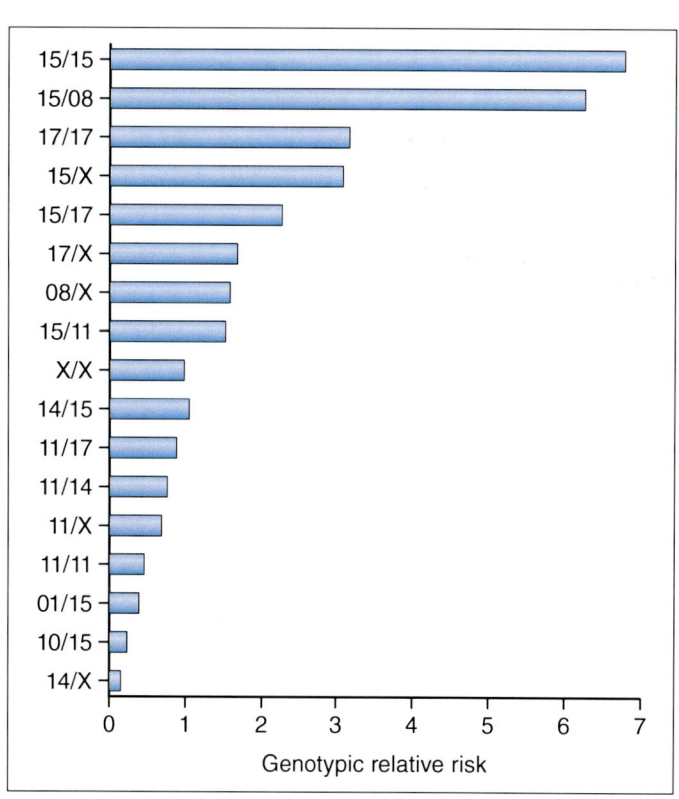

2.6 Relative risk of MS associated with different allelic combinations at *HLA-DRB1*. This figure illustrates that the risk associated with particular *HLA-DRB1* alleles can be modified by the other *HLA-DRB1* allele present. X indicates any *HLA-DRB1* allele other than those specified in the figure.[39]

Environment and MS susceptibility

Several environmental factors have been associated with risk of MS: vitamin D insufficiency, Epstein–Barr virus (EBV) infection and smoking.[24,25] These appear to act on individuals at multiple different points over the course of the lifetime (**2.7**).[26]

Vitamin D

Vitamin D is a secosteroid synthesized from cholesterol precursors by ultraviolet irradiation. An association between vitamin D levels and MS risk was suggested by the correlation between MS prevalence and ultraviolet radiation (**2.8**).[4,27,28] Similarly, vitamin D deficiency *in utero* was hypothesized as a potential cause of the month of birth effect mentioned previously (**2.3**).[13] Powerful evidence that this relationship was more than a simple association was provided by a prospective cohort study showing low vitamin D levels associated with risk of MS years before onset of disease.[29] A potential mechanism for the risk conferred by vitamin D insufficiency was identified by functional genetic studies establishing a role for vitamin D in expression of the key MS genetic risk factor, *HLA-DRB1*1501*, and binding of vitamin D receptor near genes associated with MS susceptibility.[30,31]

Epstein–Barr virus

Patients with MS are almost invariably positive for EBV antibodies (99.9%) but EBV antibody positivity is also extremely common in healthy controls (94.2%).[32] Symptomatic EBV infection or infectious mononucleosis approximately doubles the subsequent risk of MS.[33] The prevalence of infectious mononucleosis mirrors very strongly the prevalence of MS across the United Kingdom (**2.9**).[34] The precise mechanism by which EBV leads to increased MS susceptibility has not been fully established but chronic infection of B cells within the CNS and molecular mimicry have been raised as possibilities.[35]

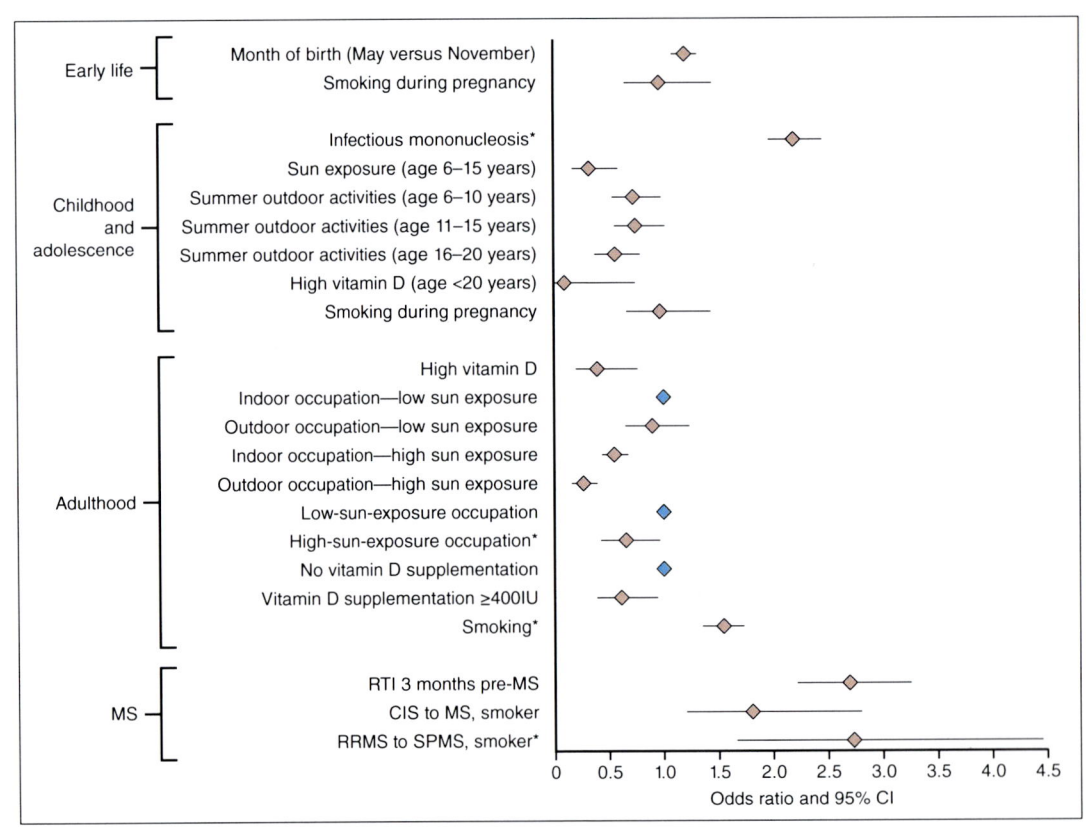

2.7 Effect size of environmental factors on MS risk during different life periods. Reference values are shown in blue. Asterisks indicate odds ratios calculated by meta-analysis that used the generic-inverse variance method and a random-effects model in Review Manager 5.0; the results were robust against changes in the model assumptions. CI, confidence intervals; CIS, clinically isolated syndrome; IU, international units; MS, multiple sclerosis; RRMS, relapsing–remitting MS; RTI, respiratory tract infection; SPMS, secondary progressive MS.[26]

Epidemiology of multiple sclerosis 13

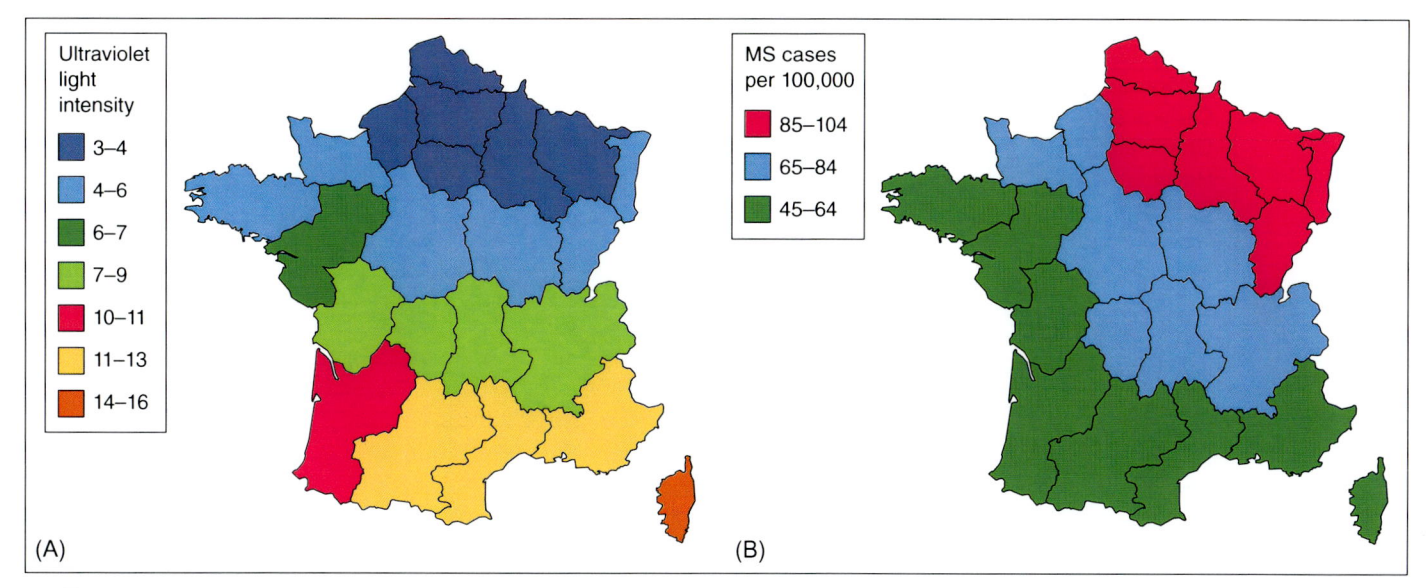

2.8 End-of-summer sunlight and MS prevalence in France. (A) End-of-summer sunlight intensity by region and (B) number of MS cases per 100 000 individuals among French farmers from the Agricole Health System.[4,26]

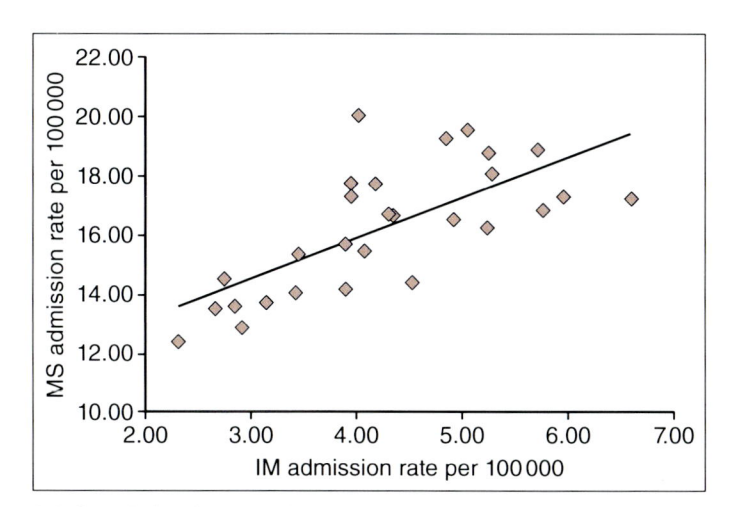

2.9 Correlation between hospitalization rates for infectious mononucleosis (IM) and MS in the United Kingdom.[34]

Smoking

Smoking cigarettes has been consistently associated with an approximately 50% increased risk of MS (**2.10**).[36] As Swedish snuff does not confer an increased susceptibility to MS, it is likely to be compounds in cigarette smoke other than nicotine that mediate the increase in MS risk.[37] The mechanism for this is currently unknown; however, it may be related to modification of antigenic proteins as has been observed in rheumatoid arthritis or by directly modulating components of the immune system.[38]

Conclusions

The epidemiology of MS is characterized by a latitude gradient of prevalence. The female-to-male sex ratio in MS is approximately 2:1 and this is increasing over time. There is a month of birth effect with spring births conferring an increased subsequent risk of MS. Susceptibility to MS is established by an interplay of multiple genetic and environmental risk factors, including vitamin D insufficiency, EBV infection and smoking.

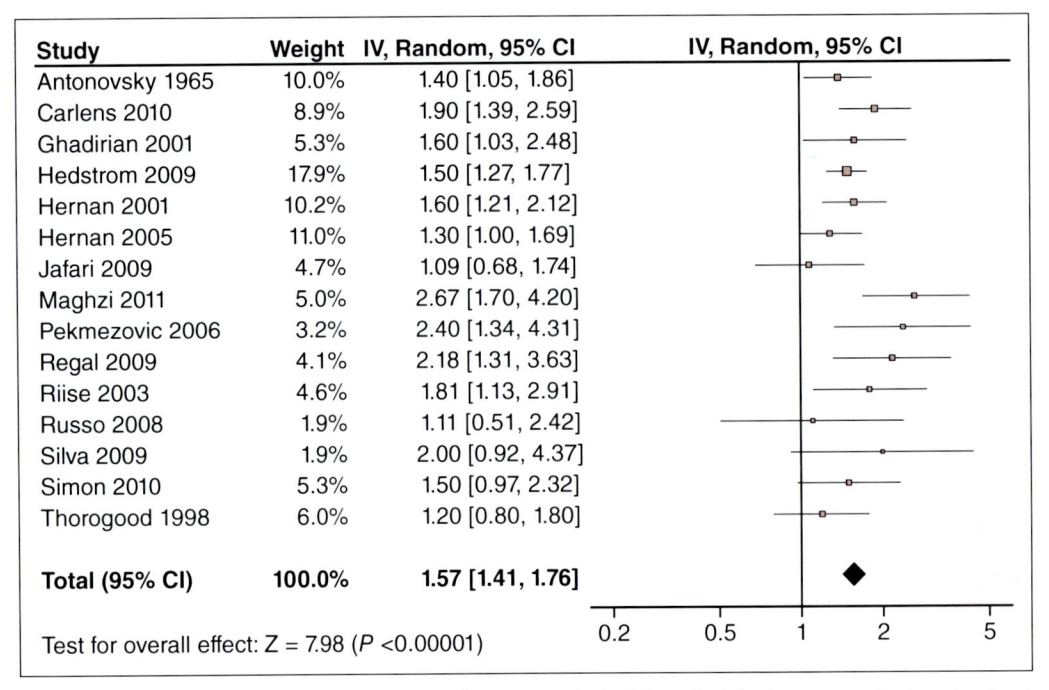

Study	Weight	IV, Random, 95% CI
Antonovsky 1965	10.0%	1.40 [1.05, 1.86]
Carlens 2010	8.9%	1.90 [1.39, 2.59]
Ghadirian 2001	5.3%	1.60 [1.03, 2.48]
Hedstrom 2009	17.9%	1.50 [1.27, 1.77]
Hernan 2001	10.2%	1.60 [1.21, 2.12]
Hernan 2005	11.0%	1.30 [1.00, 1.69]
Jafari 2009	4.7%	1.09 [0.68, 1.74]
Maghzi 2011	5.0%	2.67 [1.70, 4.20]
Pekmezovic 2006	3.2%	2.40 [1.34, 4.31]
Regal 2009	4.1%	2.18 [1.31, 3.63]
Riise 2003	4.6%	1.81 [1.13, 2.91]
Russo 2008	1.9%	1.11 [0.51, 2.42]
Silva 2009	1.9%	2.00 [0.92, 4.37]
Simon 2010	5.3%	1.50 [0.97, 2.32]
Thorogood 1998	6.0%	1.20 [0.80, 1.80]
Total (95% CI)	**100.0%**	**1.57 [1.41, 1.76]**

Test for overall effect: Z = 7.98 (P <0.00001)

2.10 Risk of MS associated with smoking. A meta-analytical forest plot of case–control and cohort studies investigating smoking and risk of MS. The total risk is displayed as a risk ratio and 95% confidence intervals. CI, confidence intervals; IV, inverse variance.[36,40]

References

1. Multiple Sclerosis International Federation. *Atlas of MS Database*. 2009. http://www.atlasofms.org/index.aspx
2. Koch-Henriksen N, Sørensen PS. The changing demographic pattern of multiple sclerosis epidemiology. *Lancet Neurol* 2010; **9**: 520–32.
3. McLeod JG, Hammond SR, Hallpike JF. Epidemiology of multiple sclerosis in Australia with NSW and SA survey results. *Med J Aust* 1994; **160**: 117–22.
4. Ebers GC. Environmental factors and multiple sclerosis. *Lancet Neurol* 2008; **7**: 268–77.
5. Handel AE, Jarvis L, McLaughlin R, Fries A, Ebers GC, Ramagopalan SV. The epidemiology of multiple sclerosis in Scotland: inferences from hospital admissions. *PLoS ONE* 2011; **6**: e14606.
6. Islam T, Gauderman WJ, Cozen W, Hamilton AS, Burnett ME, Mack TM. Differential twin concordance for multiple sclerosis by latitude of birthplace. *Ann Neurol* 2006; **60**: 56–64.
7. Noseworthy JH, Lucchinetti C, Rodriguez M, Weinshenker BG. Multiple sclerosis. *N Engl J Med* 2000; **343**: 938–52.
8. Orton SM, Herrera BM, Yee IM, et al; Canadian Collaborative Study Group. Sex ratio of multiple sclerosis in Canada: a longitudinal study. *Lancet Neurol* 2006; **5**: 932–6.
9. Alonso A, Hernán MA. Temporal trends in the incidence of multiple sclerosis: a systematic review. *Neurology* 2008; **71**: 129–35.
10. Alter M, Leibowitz U, Speer J. Risk of multiple sclerosis related to age at immigration to Israel. *Arch Neurol* 1966; **15**: 234–7.
11. Dean G, Elian M. Age at immigration to England of Asian and Caribbean immigrants and the risk of developing multiple sclerosis. *J Neurol Neurosurg Psychiatry* 1997; **63**: 565–8.
12. Hammond SR, English DR, McLeod JG. The age-range of risk of developing multiple sclerosis: evidence from a migrant population in Australia. *Brain* 2000; **123**(Pt 5): 968–74.

13. Willer CJ, Dyment DA, Sadovnick AD, et al, for the Canadian Collaborative Study Group. Timing of birth and risk of multiple sclerosis: population based study. *Br Med J* 2005; **330**: 120.
14. Staples J, Ponsonby A-L, Lim L. Low maternal exposure to ultraviolet radiation in pregnancy, month of birth, and risk of multiple sclerosis in offspring: longitudinal analysis. *Br Med J* 2010; **340**: c1640.
15. Sadovnick AD, Baird PA. The familial nature of multiple sclerosis: age-corrected empiric recurrence risks for children and siblings of patients. *Neurology* 1988; **38**: 990–1.
16. Ramagopalan SV, Dobson R, Meier UC, Giovannoni G. Multiple sclerosis: risk factors, prodromes, and potential causal pathways. *Lancet Neurol* 2010; **9**: 727–39.
17. Ebers GC, Sadovnick AD, Dyment DA, Yee IM, Willer CJ, Risch N. Parent-of-origin effect in multiple sclerosis: observations in half-siblings. *Lancet* 2004; **363**: 1773–4.
18. Hoppenbrouwers IA, Liu F, Aulchenko YS, et al. Maternal transmission of multiple sclerosis in a Dutch population. *Arch Neurol* 2008; **65**: 345–8.
19. Herrera BM, Ramagopalan SV, Lincoln MR, et al. Parent-of-origin effects in MS: observations from avuncular pairs. *Neurology* 2008; **71**: 799–803.
20. Lincoln MR, Ramagopalan SV, Chao MJ, et al. Epistasis among HLA-DRB1, HLA-DQA1, and HLA-DQB1 loci determines multiple sclerosis susceptibility. *Proc Natl Acad Sci USA* 2009; **106**: 7542–7.
21. Ramagopalan SV, Morris AP, Dyment DA, et al. The inheritance of resistance alleles in multiple sclerosis. *PLoS Genet* 2007; **3**: 1607–13.
22. Baranzini SE, Nickles D. Genetics of multiple sclerosis: swimming in an ocean of data. *Curr Opin Neurol* 2012; **25**: 239–45.
23. Ramagopalan SV, Dyment DA, Cader MZ, et al. Rare variants in the CYP27B1 gene are associated with multiple sclerosis. *Ann Neurol* 2011; **70**: 881–6.
24. Ascherio A, Munger KL. Environmental risk factors for multiple sclerosis. Part I: the role of infection. *Ann Neurol* 2007; **61**: 288–99.
25. Ascherio A, Munger KL. Environmental risk factors for multiple sclerosis. Part II: Noninfectious factors. *Ann Neurol* 2007; **61**: 504–13.
26. Handel AE, Giovannoni G, Ebers GC, Ramagopalan SV. Environmental factors and their timing in adult-onset multiple sclerosis. *Nat Rev Neurol* 2010; **6**: 156–66.
27. Handel AE, Handunnetthi L, Giovannoni G, Ebers GC, Ramagopalan SV. Genetic and environmental factors and the distribution of multiple sclerosis in Europe. *Eur J Neurol* 2010; **17**: 1210–14.
28. Ramagopalan SV, Handel AE, Giovannoni G, Rutherford Siegel S, Ebers GC, Chaplin G. Relationship of UV exposure to prevalence of multiple sclerosis in England. *Neurology* 2011; **76**: 1410–14.
29. Munger KL, Levin LI, Hollis BW, Howard NS, Ascherio A. Serum 25-hydroxyvitamin D levels and risk of multiple sclerosis. *JAMA* 2006; **296**: 2832–8.
30. Ramagopalan SV, Maugeri NJ, Handunnetthi L, et al. Expression of the multiple sclerosis-associated MHC class II allele HLA-DRB1*1501 is regulated by vitamin D. *PLoS Genet* 2009; **5**: e1000369.
31. Ramagopalan SV, Heger A, Berlanga AJ, et al. A ChIP-seq defined genome-wide map of vitamin D receptor binding: associations with disease and evolution. *Genome Res* 2010; **20**: 1352–60.
32. Goodin DS. The causal cascade to multiple sclerosis: a model for MS pathogenesis. *PLoS ONE* 2009; **4**: e4565.
33. Handel AE, Williamson AJ, Disanto G, Handunnetthi L, Giovannoni G, Ramagopalan SV. An updated meta-analysis of risk of multiple sclerosis following infectious mononucleosis. *PLoS ONE* 2010; **5:** e12496.
34. Ramagopalan SV, Hoang U, Seagroatt V, et al. Geography of hospital admissions for multiple sclerosis in England and comparison with the geography of hospital admissions for infectious mononucleosis: a descriptive study. *J Neurol Neurosurg Psychiatry* 2011; **82**: 682–7.
35. Pender MP. The essential role of Epstein-Barr virus in the pathogenesis of multiple sclerosis. *Neuroscientist* 2011; **17**: 351–67.
36. Handel AE, Williamson AJ, Disanto G, Dobson R, Giovannoni G, Ramagopalan SV. Smoking and multiple sclerosis: an updated meta-analysis. *PLoS ONE* 2011; **6**: e16149.
37. Hedström AK, Bäärnhielm M, Olsson T, Alfredsson L. Tobacco smoking, but not Swedish snuff use, increases the risk of multiple sclerosis. *Neurology* 2009; **73**: 696–701.

38. Mahdi H, Fisher BA, Källberg H, et al. Specific interaction between genotype, smoking and autoimmunity to citrullinated alpha-enolase in the etiology of rheumatoid arthritis. *Nat Genet* 2009; **41**: 1319–24.
39. Handel AE, Handunnetthi L, Ebers GC, Ramagopalan SV. Type 1 diabetes mellitus and multiple sclerosis: common etiological features. *Nat Rev Endocrinol* 2009; **5**: 655–64.
40. Handel AE, Ramagopalan SV. Smoking and multiple sclerosis: a matter of global importance. *Neuroepidemiology* 2011; **37**: 243–4.

Chapter 3

Magnetic resonance imaging in multiple sclerosis

Klaus Schmierer

Magnetic resonance imaging is the most important non-invasive tool in the diagnostic work-up of people suspected to have MS. The striking sensitivity of MRI to detect lesions in the CNS of people with MS (PwMS) was first described in 1981, shortly after MRI had become available for clinical studies.[1] MRI plays a pivotal role in the differential diagnosis of MS (Chapters 1 and 5), for treatment decisions and in clinical trials (particularly phase II).

MRI physics in a nutshell[2]

Clinical MRI makes use of the rich water content of biological tissue (or more precisely: the nuclei in hydrogen, i.e. protons) as the principal source of the signal. MRI systems create a powerful magnetic field [B_0, measured in Tesla (T)] causing the magnetic moment of protons to align along the axis of the bore called the Z axis. The protons' alignment with B_0 is not perfect though – they wobble along B_0 (similar to a gyroscope), a motion called precession (**3.1A**). When introduced into the MRI system, the sum magnetic vector (magnetization, *yellow arrow*) of protons in the body becomes aligned with B_0 (**3.1B**).

To obtain a signal that can be used to produce an image, the sum vector magnetization has to be 'pushed' out of alignment with B_0 (**3.2**). A radio-frequency wave (RF pulse) is introduced that flips the magnetization into an angle perpendicular to B_0 (**3.2B**), thereby reducing magnetization along the Z axis. As soon as the RF pulse is switched off, magnetization along the Z axis starts to build up again (longitudinal or 'T1' relaxation).

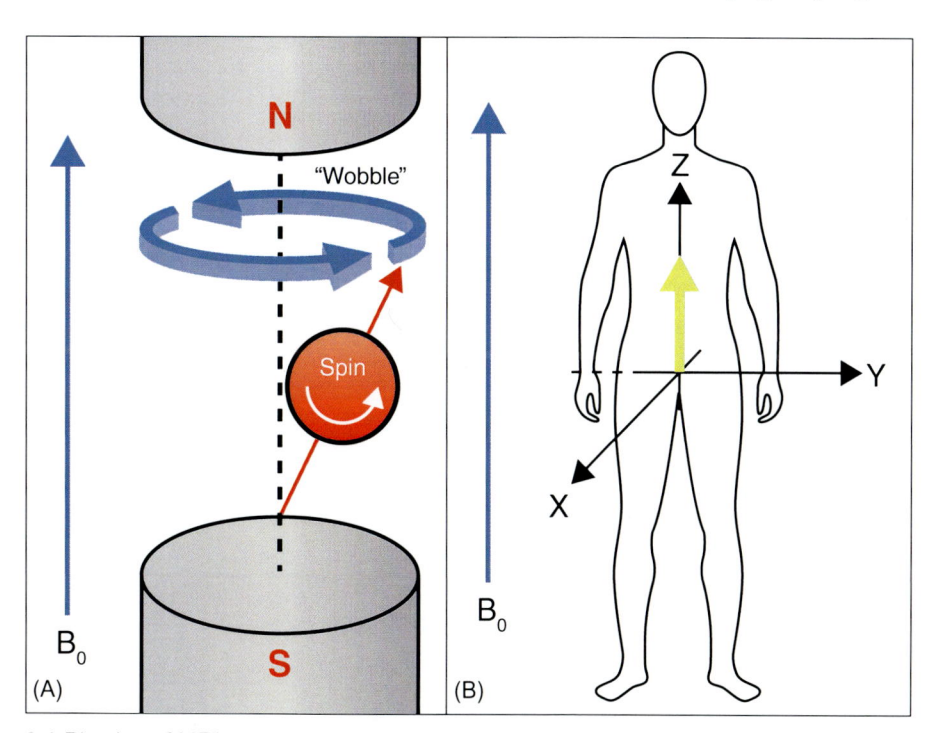

3.1 Physics of MRI.

By contrast, magnetization perpendicular to B_0 (transversal or 'T2' relaxation) is at its maximum with the RF pulse switched on and quickly decays once the RF pulse is switched off. The energy difference between the two states (with/without RF pulse) is released as an electromagnetic signal that can be detected by the receiver coil of the MRI system.

Plotting T1 and T2 against time reveals characteristic relaxation curves (**3.3**). Relaxation times (and many other MRI indices) are dependent on a number of variables, notably the proton content of the tissue examined, thereby providing a basis for the contrast detection of differences between 'normal' and 'pathologic'.

MRI in the diagnosis of MS

Lesions detected on MRI were incorporated for the first time as evidence of dissemination in time and space in

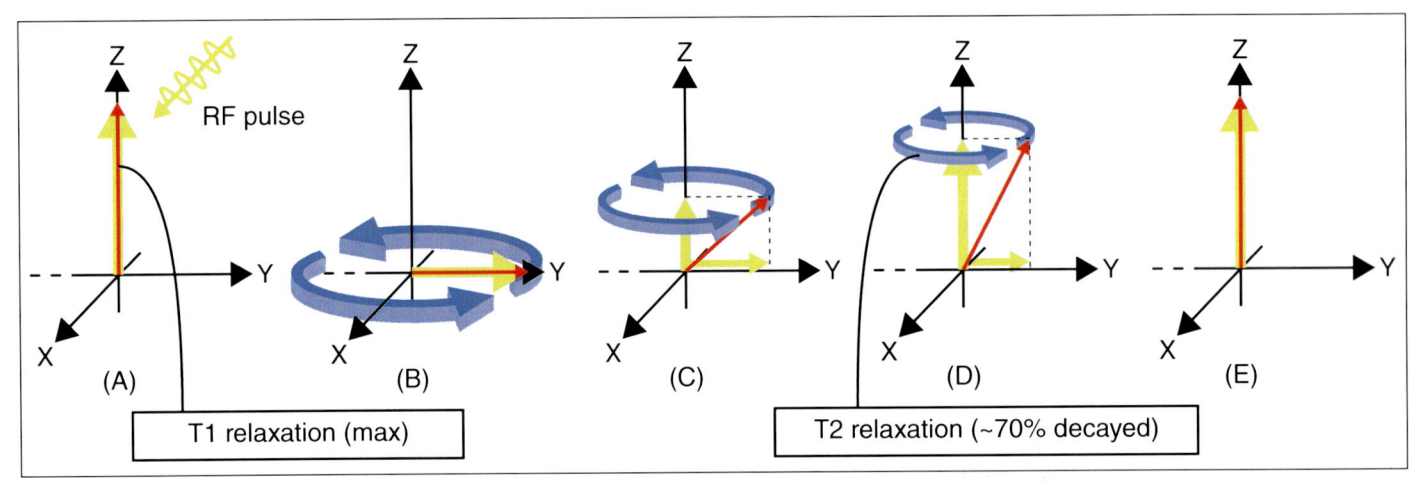

3.2 Diagrammatic representation of the production of the electromagnetic signal that is detected by the receiver coil of the MRI system.

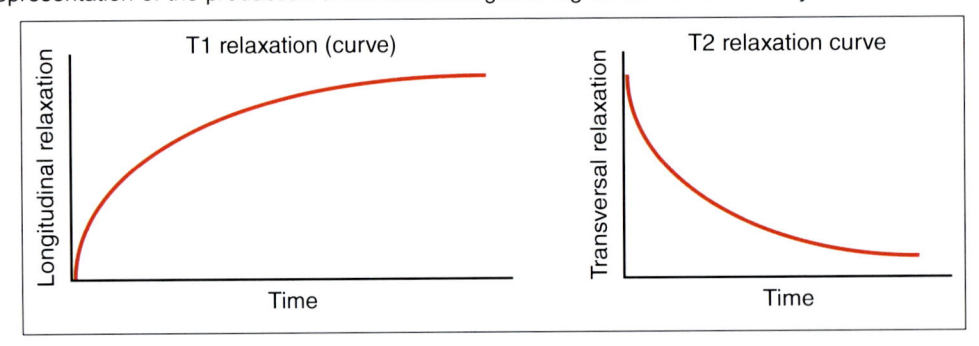

3.3 T1 and T2 relaxation curves.

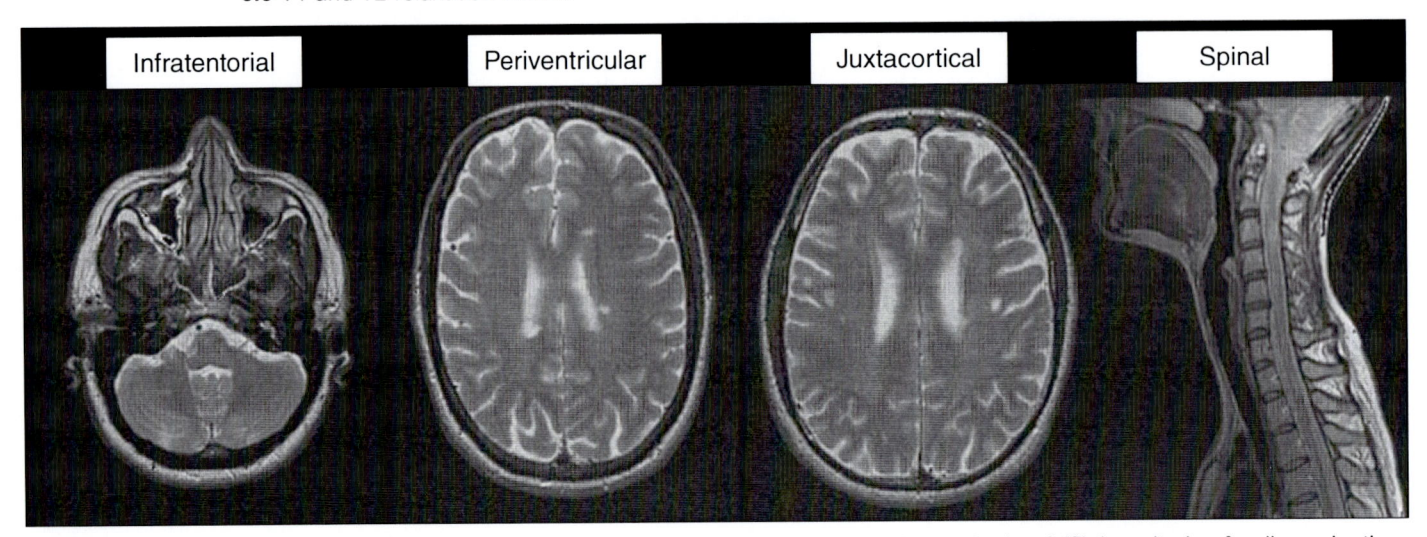

3.4 Key locations of lesions on T2-weighted MRI. At least one lesion in two locations is required to fulfil the criterion for dissemination in space.[5]

the 1982 review of diagnostic criteria for MS.[3] However, it took another 18 years for MRI to obtain its current role in the early diagnosis of MS, enabling a diagnosis to be made with high accuracy even in the absence of a second *clinical* event of demyelination. The most recent (2011) update of the so-called 'McDonald criteria' incorporates lesions in four key locations of the CNS to show evidence for dissemination in space (**3.4**). Dissemination in time criteria on MRI can be fulfilled by either (a) occurrence of a new lesion on T2-weighted and/or gadolinium-enhanced follow-up MRI, or (b) the simultaneous presence of asymptomatic gadolinium-enhancing (Gd+) and non-enhancing lesions (**3.5**).[4]

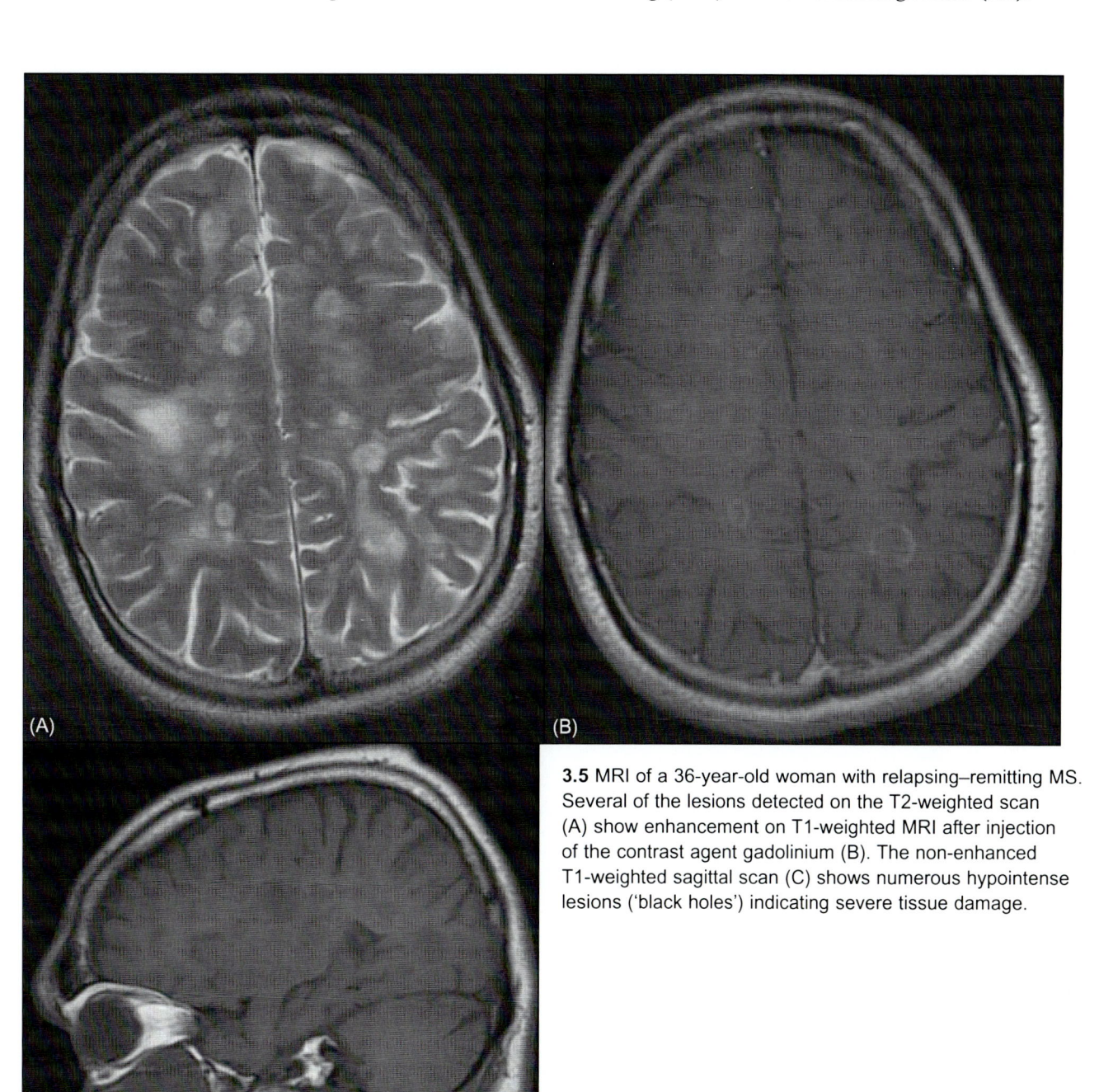

3.5 MRI of a 36-year-old woman with relapsing–remitting MS. Several of the lesions detected on the T2-weighted scan (A) show enhancement on T1-weighted MRI after injection of the contrast agent gadolinium (B). The non-enhanced T1-weighted sagittal scan (C) shows numerous hypointense lesions ('black holes') indicating severe tissue damage.

MRI as a tool for prognosis and treatment decisions

The number of lesions suggestive of demyelination detected on brain MRI at first clinical presentation can give an indication of future disease course. *Table 3.1* shows number (*n*) of lesions and clinical status in a cohort of 107 people followed up over 20 years after their first presentation with a clinically isolated syndrome of demyelination.[6] Prognostic information obtained using MRI plays an ever more important role in the clinical management of PwMS. While detection of new lesions on MRI is an established eligibility criterion (in the UK) for treatment with both natalizumab and (the small cohort of PwMS treated with) mitoxantrone, the predictive value of MRI for other disease-modifying treatments, such as the β-interferons is becoming increasingly well defined.[7,8]

MRI in clinical trials of MS

Clinical trials involving PwMS are virtually unthinkable without MRI as one of several (if not the major) tools to assess outcome. In particular, phase II trials have benefited from manageable sample sizes observed over a limited period of time (usually 6 months on treatment) when MRI measures are being used to assess outcome. Box 3.1 provides an overview of MRI indices commonly used in clinical trials, such as the number and/or size of new lesions on T2-weighted MRI, lesion severity ('black holes' on T1-weighted scans) and brain atrophy (**3.5, 3.6**). In **3.7** the results are shown from an exemplary trial in which Gd+ lesions (here the mean total number of all Gd+ lesions combined on MRI scans obtained at weeks 12, 16, 20 and 24) were used to assess outcome.

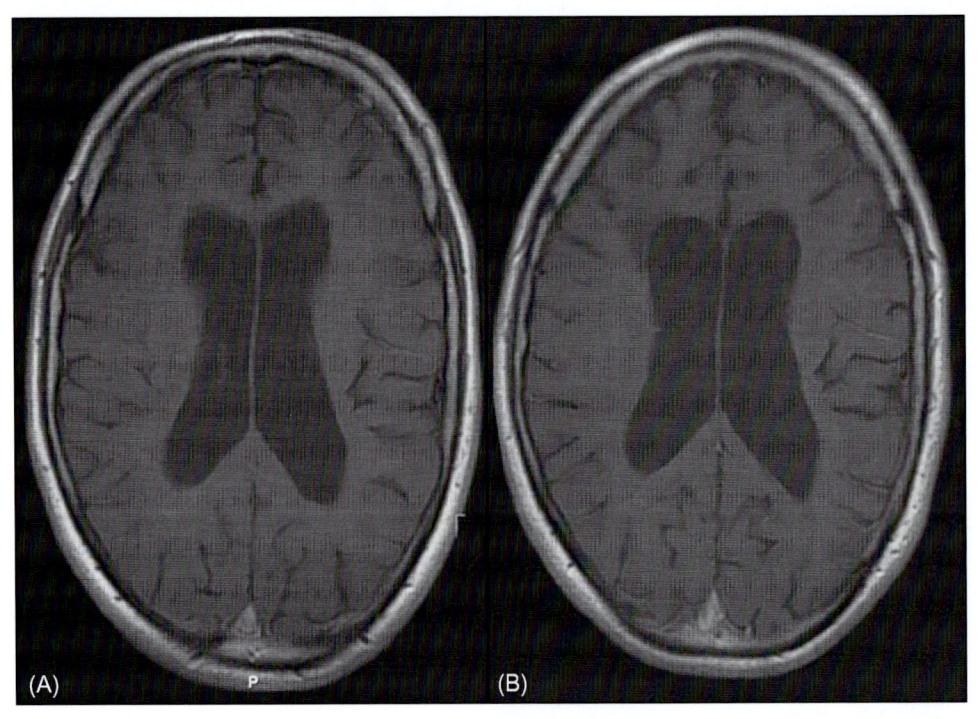

Table 3.1 Cohort 20-year follow up study[6]

	n lesions on T2-weighted MRI at baseline			
	0	1–3	4–9	≥10
n CIS at 20 years	79%	18%	15%	19%
n PwMS at 20 years	21%	82%	85%	81%
n PwMS with EDSS > 3 at 20 years	26%	36%	50%	65%
n PwMS with EDSS ≥ 6 at 20 years	6%	18%	35%	45%

CIS, clincially isolated syndrome; EDSS, Expanded Disability Status Scale; PwMS, people with MS.

3.6 T1-weighted MRI of a 41-year-old man with severe relapsing–remitting MS (A), and follow-up scan 2 years later (B). Comparison of the two scans suggests enlargement of the lateral ventricles as a result of brain atrophy.

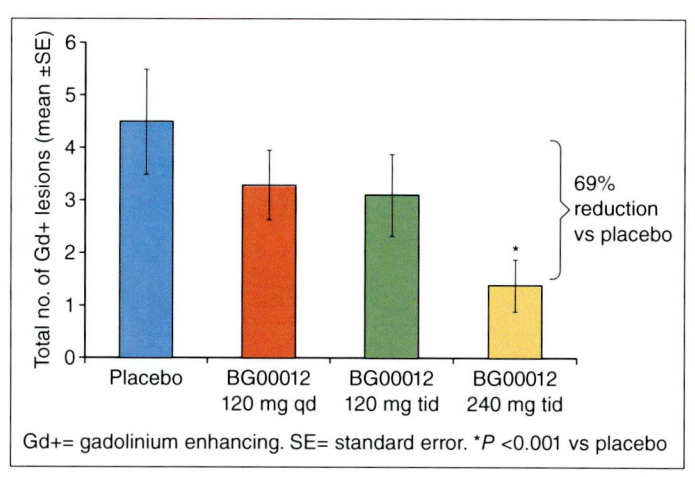

3.7 The total number of Gd-enhancing lesions can be a useful outcome measure in the MS clinical trials.

The future of MRI in MS

Major shortcomings of current MRI techniques include the lack of (a) sensitivity for lesions affecting CNS grey matter, and (b) specificity for tissue components most relevant in the pathophysiology of MS (neurons, axons, inflammatory and glial cells), and their physiological state (e.g. energy failure). These limitations are likely to be overcome through the increased availability of MRI systems operating at higher field strength (3T and beyond; **3.8**);[10] further improvements in hardware technology (e.g. multiarray receive coils); the translation of quantitative techniques (e.g. diffusion tensor, magnetization transfer, short T2- and susceptibility-weighted imaging); and faster, simpler post-processing algorithms.[11]

Box 3.1 Overview of MRI indices commonly used in clinical trials

MRI measures of disease in MS clinical trials

- Total lesion number on T2-weighted MRI; as these T2 lesions mostly reflect demyelination and tend not to disappear (even when partial remyelination occurs), their overall number indicates the total burden of disease since onset.

- Active lesions, i.e. either (i) Gd+ lesions, or (ii) new lesions that occur between two successive T2-weighted scans. Gd+ and new T2 lesions are collectively referred to as 'combined unique active lesions'.

- Chronic black holes, which comprise a subset of T2 lesions with a persistently low signal (hypointensity) on T1-weighted MRI, represent lesions with considerable axonal damage and expanded extracellular spaces; they should be distinguished from temporary hypointensity around the time of lesion development and Gd enhancement.

- Brain atrophy is inferred from brain volume shrinkage, which is most readily measured from sequential T1-weighted MRI before Gd administration, using segmentation-based and/or registration-based analysis techniques that determine brain volume changes over time. Temporary brain volume loss due to water shifts, termed 'pseudoatrophy', can be observed after alcohol intake, and use of steroids and other anti-inflammatory drugs.

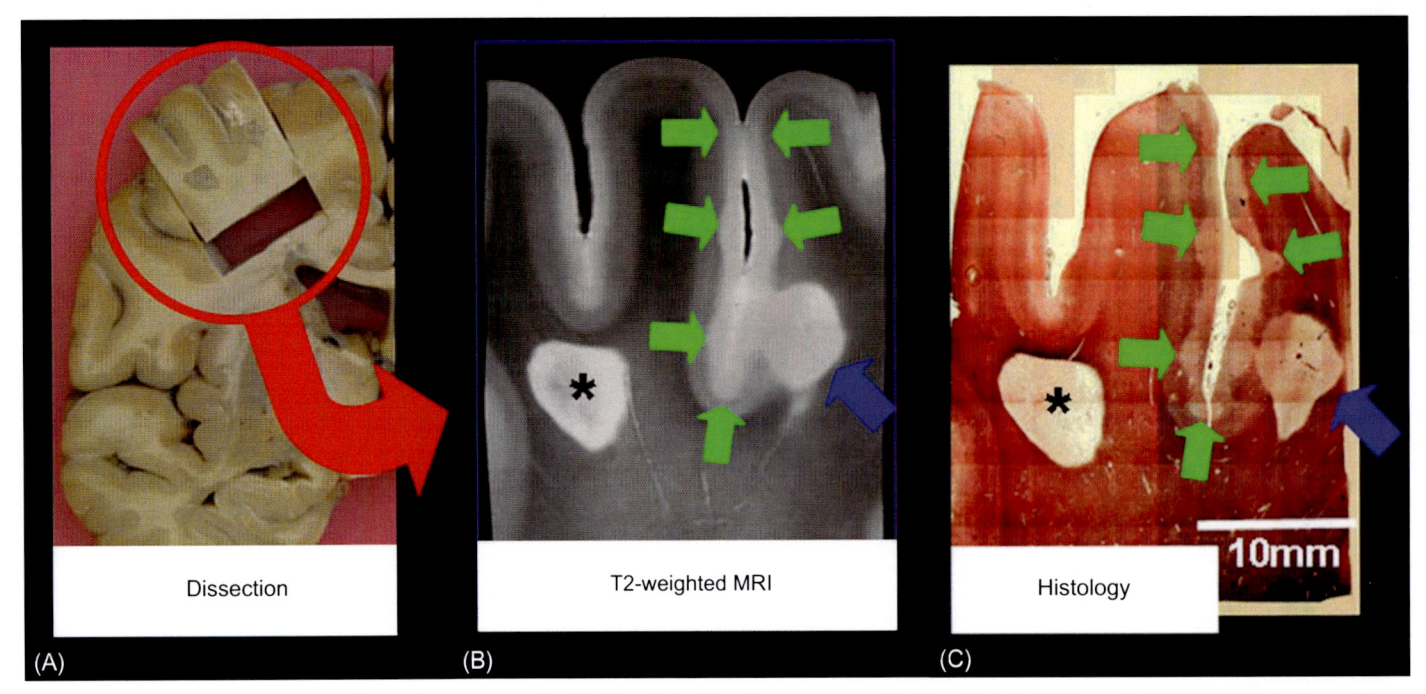

3.8 Post mortem MS brain scanning to improve cortical lesion detection (*green arrows*) using high field (here: 9.4T) MRI. After dissection, tissue blocks (A) are scanned (B) and subsequently processed for histology (here: immunostained for myelin basic protein) (C). *Blue arrows* indicate white matter component of a mixed (grey/white matter) lesion. Asterisks indicate a lesion affecting white matter only.

References

1. Young IR, Hall AS, Pallis CA, Legg NJ, Bydder GM, Steiner RE. Nuclear magnetic resonance imaging of the brain in multiple sclerosis. *Lancet* 1981; **14**: 1063–6.
2. Schild HH. *MRI Made Easy – well almost*. Berlin: Nationales Druckhaus 1990.
3. Poser CM, Paty DW, Scheinberg L, et al. New diagnostic criteria for multiple sclerosis: guidelines for research protocols. *Ann Neurol* 1983; **13**: 227–31.
4. Polman CH, Reingold SC, Banwell B, et al. Diagnostic Criteria for Multiple Sclerosis: 2010 Revisions to the McDonald Criteria. *Ann Neurol* 2011; **69**: 292–302.
5. Swanton JK, Rovira A, Tintore M, et al. MRI criteria for multiple sclerosis in patients presenting with clinically isolated syndromes: a multicentre retrospective study. *Lancet Neurol* 2007; **6**: 677–86.
6. Fisniku LK, Brex PA, Altmann DR, et al. Disability and T2 MRI lesions: a 20-year follow-up of patients with relapse onset of multiple sclerosis. *Brain* 2008; **131**: 808–17.
7. Rudick RA, Polman CH. Current approaches to the identification and management of breakthrough disease in patients with multiple sclerosis. *Lancet Neurol* 2009; **8**: 545–59.
8. Sormani MP, Stubinski B, Cornelisse P, Rocak S, Li D, De Stefano N. Magnetic resonance active lesions as individual-level surrogate for relapses in multiple sclerosis. *Mult Scler* 2011; **17**: 541–9.
9. Kappos L, Gold R, Miller DH, et al; BG-12 Phase IIb Study Investigators. Efficacy and safety of oral fumarate in patients with relapsing-remitting multiple sclerosis: a multicentre, randomised, double-blind, placebo-controlled phase IIb study. *Lancet* 2008; **372**: 1463–72.
10. Schmierer K, Parkes HG, So PW, et al. High field (9.4 Tesla) magnetic resonance imaging of cortical grey matter lesions in multiple sclerosis. *Brain* 2010; **133**: 858–67.
11. Filippi M, Rocca MA, De Stefano N, et al. Magnetic resonance techniques in multiple sclerosis: the present and the future. *Arch Neurol* 2011; **68**: 1514–20.

Chapter 4

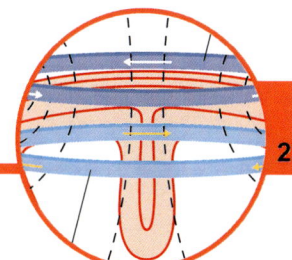

Neurophysiology of multiple sclerosis

Mark Baker and Cecilia Blomberg

The physiology of myelin

One of the major functions of myelin, certainly in the periphery, is to increase impulse conduction velocity.[1] However, in central myelinated axons, because most of them are so small (with submicron diameters), the provision of a sheath is not expected to increase conduction velocity so dramatically.[2] A myelin sheath also reduces the energy expenditure per impulse by creating a conducting structure that has a low electrical capacity.[3,4] Axons express a variety of transmembrane voltage-gated ion channels, but the sodium channels are essential for excitability, which harnesses the sodium ion electrochemical gradient across the membrane to generate the impulse upswing. Sodium channels are voltage-gated and activated by depolarization. Sodium channels are found at high density at nodes of Ranvier (estimated as near to $1000/\mu m^2$),[5] but at very low density in the axolemma under the myelin, which means that, normally, excitability is confined to nodes of Ranvier (e.g. reference 6), and the internodes are inexcitable. This distribution of sodium channels arises during development,[7] through interactions between the axon and enveloping myelinating cell.[8] Impulse conduction in all axons depends upon the flow of local circuit current (**4.1**). The local circuit provides a mechanism for membrane actively generating the impulse to depolarize the neighbouring region, and in so doing to recruit sodium channels. With an intact myelin sheath, local circuit current can spread further than if it were not present, allowing the sequential recruitment of nodes of Ranvier to impulse propagation and saltatory conduction. Loss of myelin therefore impacts impulse conduction profoundly. It can give rise to complete conduction failure, intermittent conduction failure (where propagation becomes activity or impulse frequency dependent), temperature-dependent deficits (Uhthoff's phenomenon), and impulse conduction

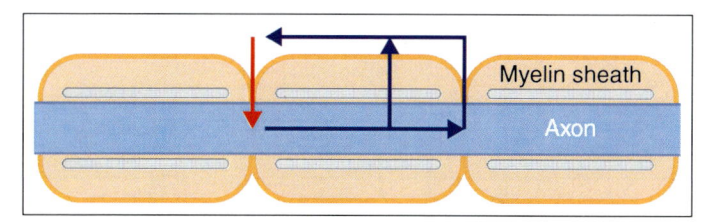

4.1 Local circuit current flow allows impulse propagation in a nerve. The *red arrow* indicates ionic sodium current at an active node of Ranvier, and the *blue arrows* indicate longitudinal and radial local circuit current, depolarizing the next node and recruiting it to the impulse. The impulse is conducted from left to right.

slowing, depending upon severity of the loss and degree to which functional recovery may be able to take place (including remyelination). In contrast, permanent disability gradually accruing during the progressive phase of MS is now attributed largely to the death of axons, producing an irreversible functional deficit.

Experimental studies have revealed that the loss of myelin and subsequent acute conduction failure can be followed several days later by a restoration of function brought about by the formation of a new distribution of sodium channels.[6] This new distribution can allow continuous conduction across a denuded internode, albeit with a substantially reduced conduction velocity (**4.2**). This finding, not only revealing an impressive capacity of nerves to compensate for the loss of myelin, has been considered to be key in providing an explanation for the delays in evoked potential latency brought about by MS.

Central axons and demyelination

While holding features in common,[8,9] central myelinated axons differ from peripheral myelinated axons in important ways. Central axons are associated with two types of glial cells: oligodendrocytes and astrocytes. Oligodendrocytes

24 Neurophysiology of multiple sclerosis

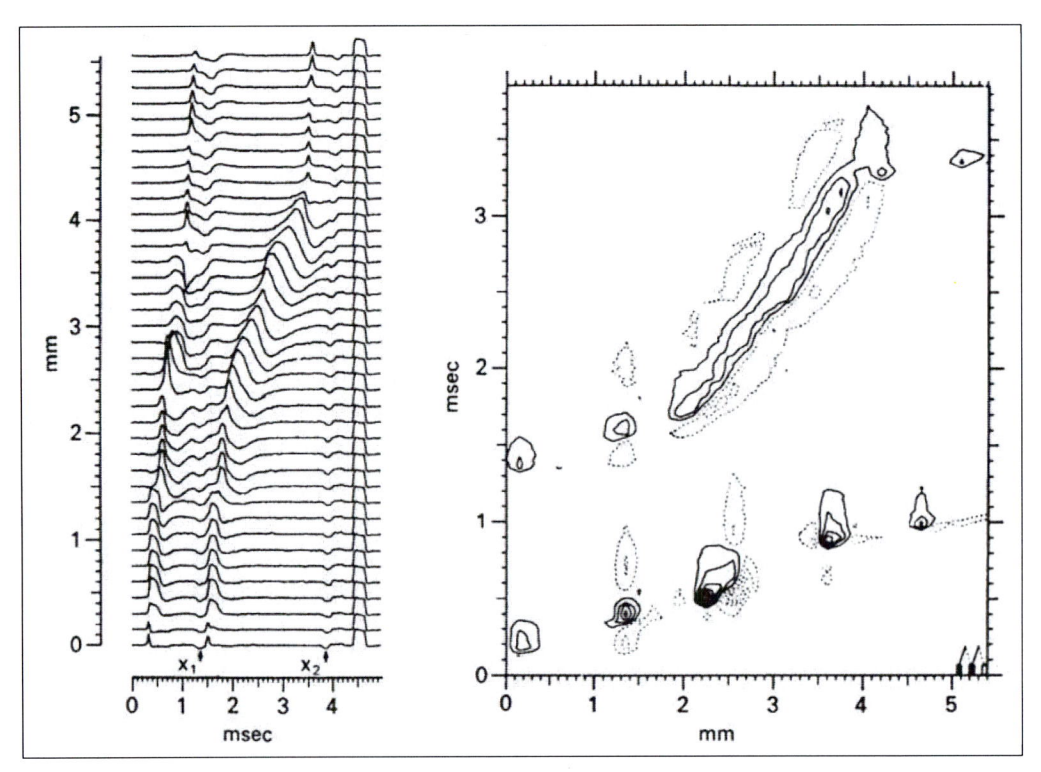

4.2 Continuous conduction in an acutely demyelinated peripheral nerve 14 days after exposure to diphtheria toxin. The region of continuous conduction is clearly apparent in the radial current density contour map as the region with the greatest slope in the time/distance plot. (From Bostock and Sears. The internodal axon membrane: electrical excitability and continuous conduction in segmental demyelination. *J Physiol* 1978; **280**: 273–301.)

provide myelin sheaths, while astrocyte processes make close contact at central nodes.[9] Peripheral axons are myelinated by Schwann cells, and CNS and peripheral nervous system myelin structural integrity is maintained by different proteins that also provide selective immunogenic epitopes, including P0 in the periphery and myelin basic protein in the CNS. Most central myelinated axons are submicron in diameter, and nerve fibres so small would be unmyelinated if they were operating in the periphery. While it is likely that an unmyelinated axon (employing continuous conduction) of similar submicron diameter would conduct a little more slowly than one enveloped by myelin, the difference in conduction velocity is predicted to be less than an order of magnitude;[2] this is because in a tiny myelinated axon, the nodes of Ranvier must be close together, owing to the biophysical constraint of a short length constant. Following central demyelination, there is evidence that some restoration of function is probably afforded by remyelination within demyelinated regions to form 'shadow plaques',[10] but there is good evidence for a slowing of impulse progression that persists in patients and has been measured using visual evoked potentials (VEPs).[11,12]

Clinical applications

Neurophysiological tests assess functional changes within the nervous system, and evoked potentials can provide evidence of damage within specific CNS tracts. With the advent of MRI, neurophysiology is less often used in the diagnosis of MS. However, evoked potential tests can identify small lesions or clinically silent lesions and thereby improve diagnosis by identifying multiple lesions, even if these are not apparent clinically or on imaging.

Different evoked potentials test the function of different neurological tracts. Abnormalities of evoked potentials are not specific for particular pathological conditions and so the findings must be interpreted within the clinical context. It is important to remember that target organ damage such as peripheral nerve disease and retinal disease can also cause abnormal results without there necessarily being any involvement of the CNS.

In simple terms, a delay in the latency of potentials is indicative of reduced conduction velocity secondary to demyelination and reduced amplitude of potentials reflects complete conduction block or axonal damage.

Of the evoked potential tests commonly used in clinical practice, VEPs are the most useful to identify clinically silent lesions.[13]

Visual evoked potentials

Pattern VEPs measure the response from the occipital cortex generated when the eye is presented with an alternating chequerboard pattern (**4.3**). Each eye is tested separately and the signal recorded using electrodes across the back of the head.

In a normal study there is an initial negative peak at approximately 75 msecs (N75) followed by a positive peak at 100 msec (P100) and a negative peak at 135 msec (N135) (**4.4**). The latency of the VEP is measured at P100, which shows relatively little variation between subjects and over time.[14]

Optic neuritis is the presenting manifestation of MS in 15–20% of patients[15–17] and occurs at some point in the course of disease in 50–66% of patients.[18,19] However, 90% of patients have evidence of optic nerve involvement on VEPs.[11]

The pattern of changes seen in VEP following optic neuritis start with a marked reduction in VEP amplitude within the first few days following the onset of symptoms (**4.5**),[20] which is thought to be due to oedema of the optic nerve related to the acute inflammatory response. The marked loss of VEP amplitude during the acute phase tends to improve over a few weeks. There is an improvement in VEP amplitude accompanied by an increase in VEP latency, which is thought to reflect reduced conduction velocity secondary to demyelination of the optic nerve[21–23] (**4.6**). The delay in VEP tends to persist for months or years despite good functional recovery but sometimes the latency recovers to near normal.[24]

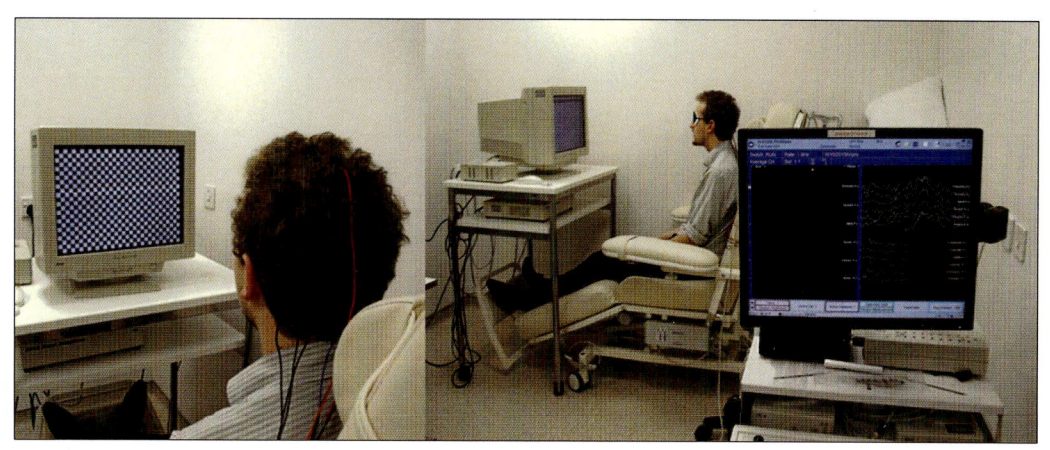

4.3 Recording of a pattern visual evoked potential.

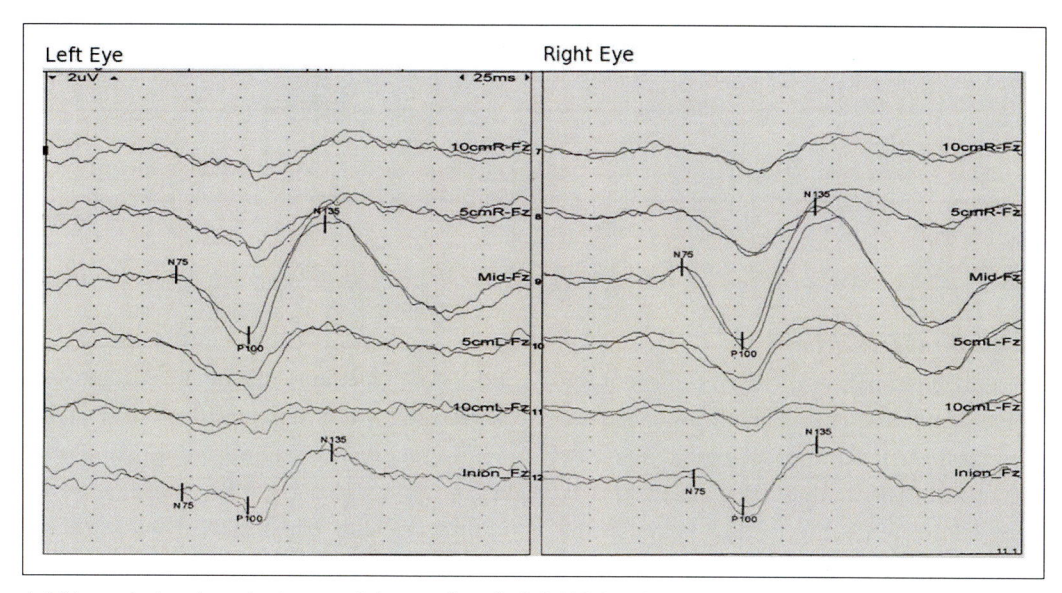

4.4 Normal visual evoked potential recording (left P100 is 105 msec, right P100 is 104 msec). (Image courtesy of Richard Pottinger.)

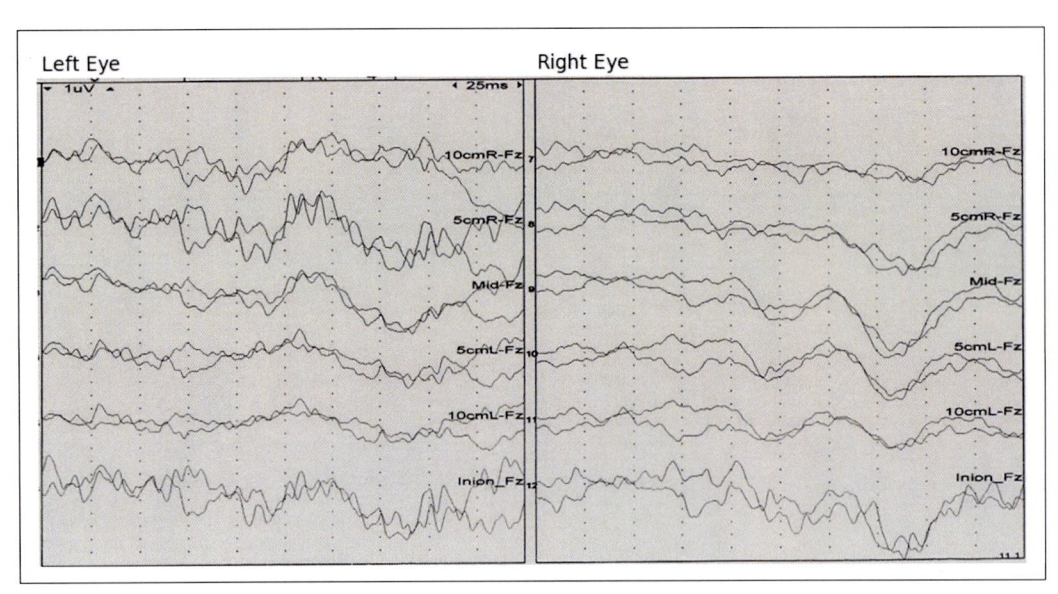

4.5 Visual evoked potential recording with no clear, measurable responses (note that the sensitivity of the traces is increased). (Image courtesy of Richard Pottinger.)

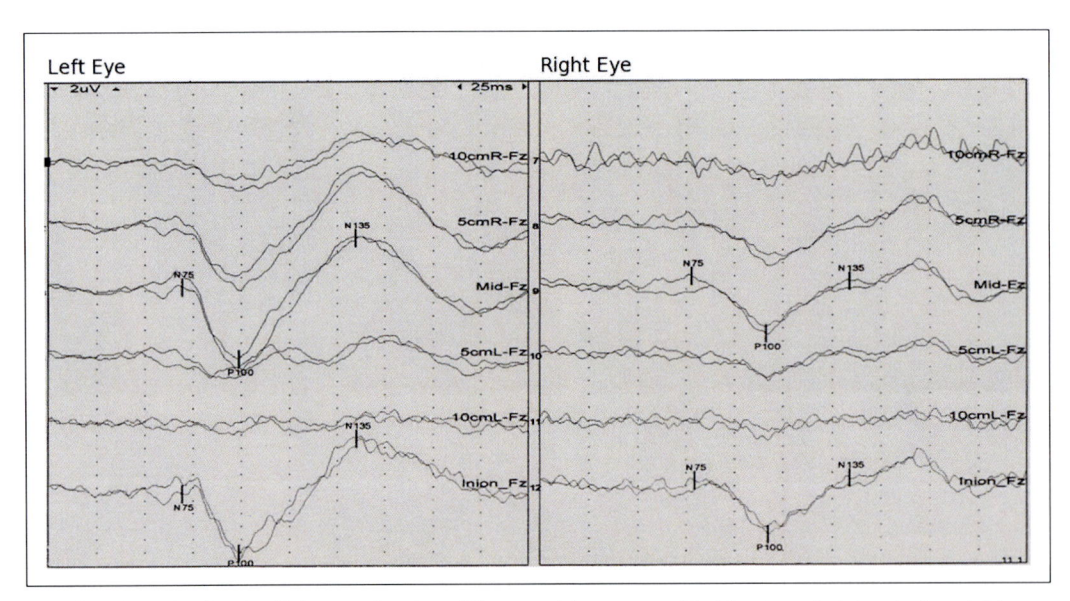

4.6 Visual evoked potential recording in a 24-year-old woman with blurring of vision in the right eye 2 years ago. The right P100 latency is increased at 116 msec. Left P100 latency is normal at 99 msec. (Image courtesy of Richard Pottinger.)

Somatosensory evoked potentials

Somatosensory evoked potentials (SSEPs) are recorded from peripheral nerve, spine and cortex following electrical stimulation of a nerve distally. The stimulus used predominantly activates large diameter, fast conducting fibres (Aα and Aβ). The most commonly stimulated is the median nerve in the upper limb and tibial nerve in the lower limb. The response is predominantly mediated via the dorsal columns.[25,26]

Latency, amplitude and side-to-side comparisons can be made and various peaks can be measured but P40 (tibial) and N20 (median) from the somatosensory cortex are diagnostically the most useful peaks[27] (**4.7**).

The incidence of abnormalities in patients with definite MS is approximately 80%[27] and abnormalities are most often seen with SSEPs recorded with stimulation of the lower limbs.[28] SSEPs can detect subclinical lesions and are abnormal in approximately one-third of patients with MS without clinical involvement of somatosensory pathways.[29]

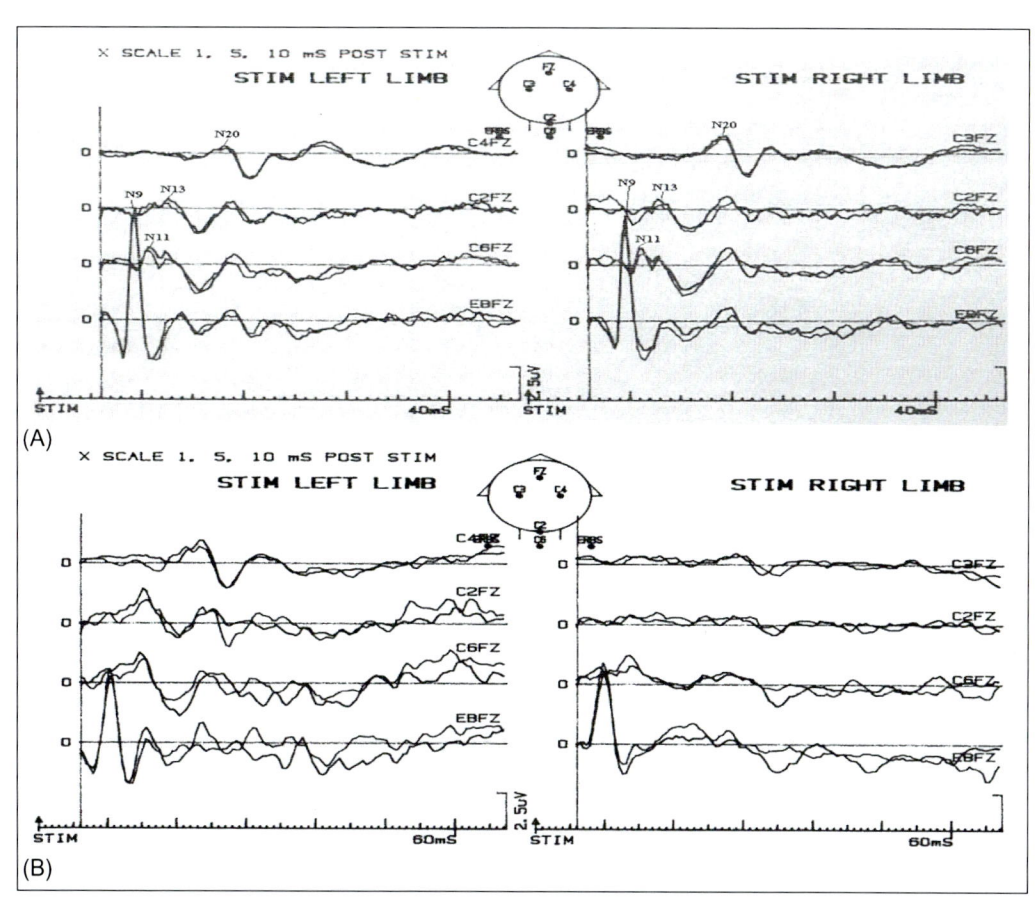

4.7 (A) Normal median somatosensory evoked potentials (right N20 is 19 msec, left N20 is 18 msec). (B) Median somatosensory evoked potentials in a 24-year-old woman with 6-week history of tingling in the right hand and weakness of the right arm. The right N20 is of reduced amplitude and delayed but N9 (peripheral response from right Erb's point) is normal (right N20 is 28 msec, left N20 is 18 msec). (Image courtesy of Richard Pottinger.)

Motor evoked potentials

In single pulse transcranial magnetic stimulation, a brief, high-current pulse is passed through a coil generating a magnetic field, which induces an electrical field in the brain (**4.8, 4.9**). When the coil is placed over the motor cortex, contraction of the target muscle occurs. From this, the motor tracts can be assessed and central motor conduction time (CMCT) can be recorded and subclinical corticospinal tract lesions may be identified. CMCT is usually measured with the target muscle voluntarily contracting, which gives the shortest latency.[30]

Various abnormalities of motor evoked potentials are seen in MS but increased CMCT is the most common[31] (**4.10**). CMCT is prolonged in 56–93% of patients with definite MS. Sensitivity is increased if lower limb muscles are tested and abnormalities are more common in progressive rather than relapsing–remitting MS.[30]

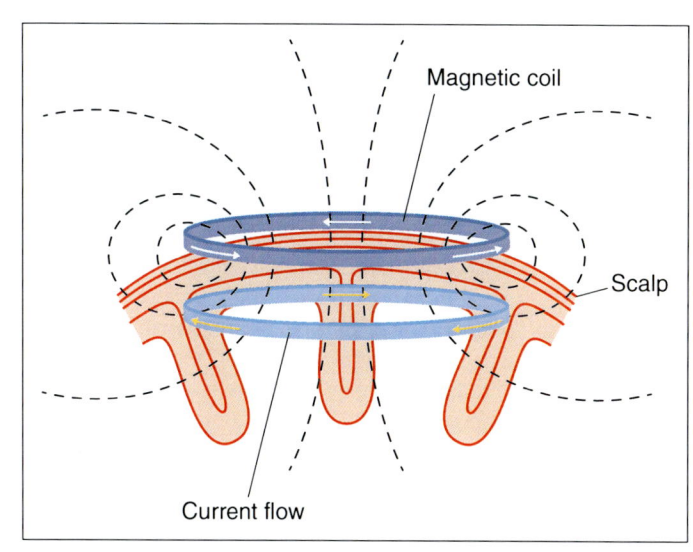

4.8 Diagramatic representation of magnetic and electrical field induced by single pulse transcranial magnetic stimulation (From Hallell M. Transcranial magnetic stimulation and the human brain. *Nature* 2000; **406**: 147–50.)

28 Neurophysiology of multiple sclerosis

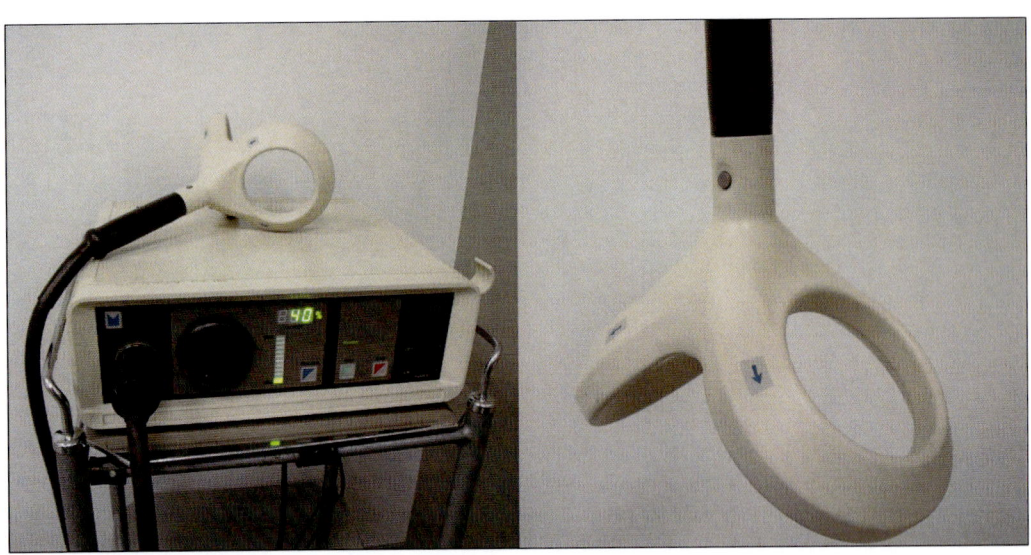

4.9 Magstim 200 magnetic stimulator with a 'figure-of-eight' coil. The maximum stimulation occurs under the intersection.

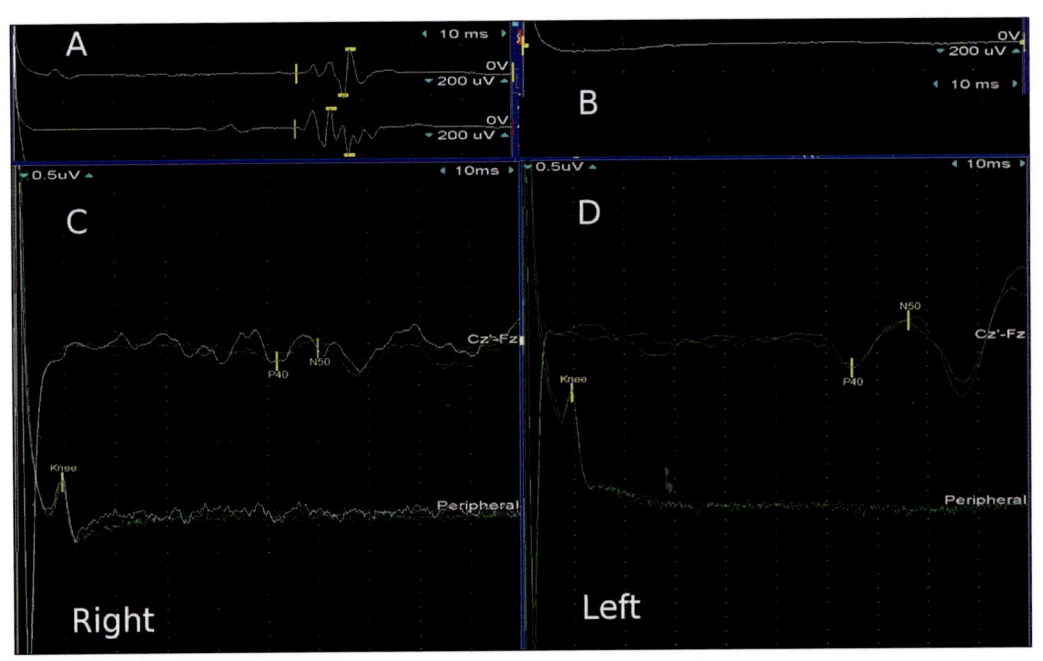

4.10 A 58-year-old man with history of weakness and parasthesiae of the lower limbs. MRI showed inflammatory cord lesions in the cervical and thoracic spine. (A,B) Motor evoked potentials from abductor hallucis. No clear response was generated on the left and the response on the right was markedly delayed at 50.7 msec (central motor conduction time 29.0 msec). (C,D) Tibials somatosensory evoked potentials from the same patient showing markedly delayed cortical responses (right P40 is 51.8; left P40 is 64.9).

Brainstem auditory evoked potentials

Brainstem auditory evoked potentials (BAEPs) are recorded from the scalp over the vertex and occur in response to auditory stimuli in the form of clicks, which are presented several times per second. The evoked response consists of five main waveforms, which represent different anatomical structures of the VIIIth cranial nerve and brainstem (*Table 4.1*).

Neurophysiology of multiple sclerosis

Table 4.1 Summary of generators for the main waveforms of the brainstem auditory evoked potential[32]

Wave number	Generator
I	VIII nerve
II	Cochlear nucleus
III	Superior olivary complex
IV/V	Lateral lemniscus/inferior colliculi

In MS, wave I should be preserved (in the absence of unrelated peripheral auditory disease) and the most common abnormality is reduction or absence of wave V[32] (**4.11**). The diagnostic yield of BAEPs is lower than SSEPs and VEPs[33,34] and the American Academy of Neurology advises that there is insufficient evidence to recommend using BAEPs to identify patients at increased risk for developing clinically definite MS.[13]

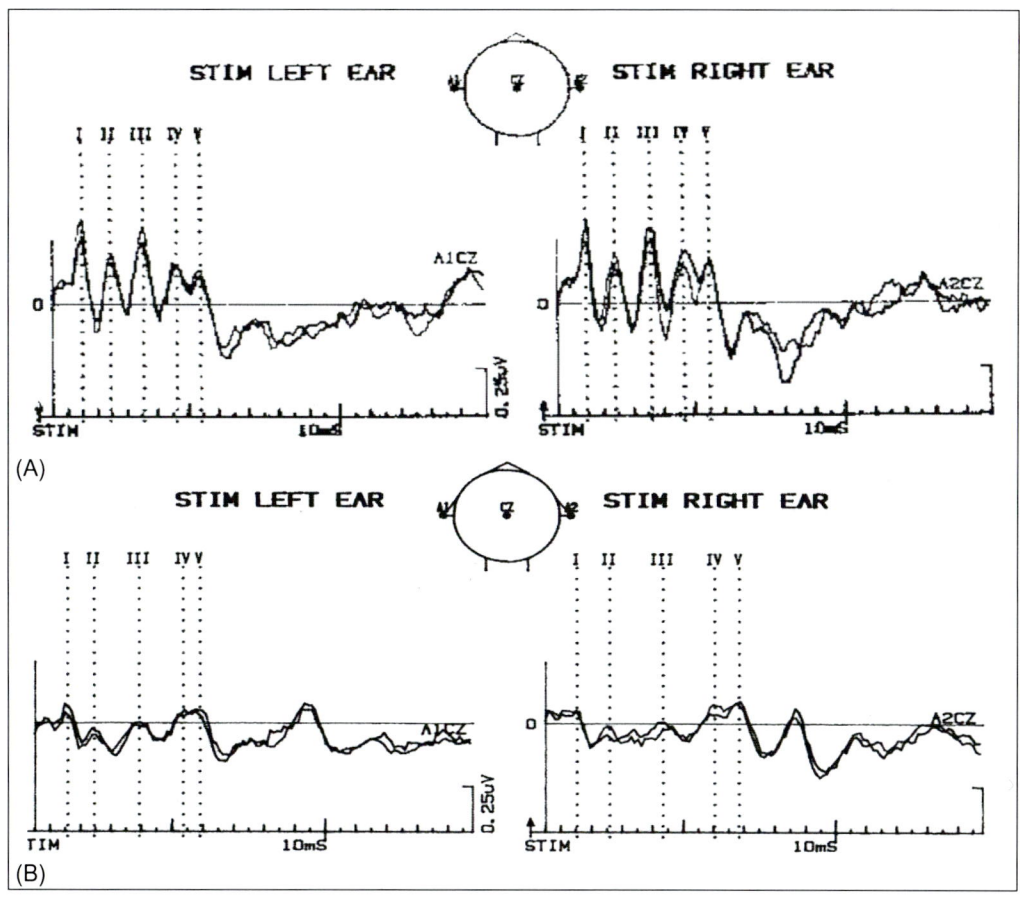

4.11 (A) Brainstem auditory evoked potentials in a normal subject. (B) Brainstem auditory evoked potentials in a patient with MS showing increased latency of right wave V (right wave V latency is 6.9 msec; left wave V latency is 5.9 msec). (Image courtesy of Richard Pottinger.)

References

1. Rushton WAH. A theory of the effects of fibre size in medulated nerve. *J Physiol* 1951; **115**: 101–22.
2. Perge JA, Koch K, Miller R, Sterling P, Balasubramanian V. How the optic nerve allocates space, energy capacity, and information. *J Neurosci* 2009; **29**: 7917–28.
3. Barrett EF, Barrett JN. Intracellular recording from vertebrate myelinated axons: mechanism of the depolarizing afterpotential. *J Physiol* 1982; **323**: 117–44.
4. Baker MD. Axonal flip-flops and oscillators. *TINS* 2000; **23**: 514–19.
5. Waxman SG, Ritchie JM. Molecular dissection of the myelinated axon. *Ann Neurol* 1993; **33**: 121–36.

6. Bostock H, Sears TA, Sherratt RM. The spatial distribution of excitability and membrane current in normal and demyelinated mammalian nerve fibres. *J Physiol* 1983; **341**: 41–58.
7. Rasband MN, Shrager P. Ion channel sequestration in central nervous system axons. *J Physiol* 2000; **525**: 63–73.
8. Poliak S, Peles E. Local differentiation of myelinated axons at nodes of Ranvier. *Nat Rev Neurosci* 2003; **4**: 968–80.
9. Hildebrand C, Mohseni S. The structure of myeliated axons in the CNS. In: Waxman SG (ed.) *Multiple Sclerosis as a Neuronal Disease*. Waltham, MA: Academic Press Inc., 2005: 1–28.
10. Keirstead HS, Blakemore WF. The role of oligodendrocytes and oligodendrocyte progenitors in CNS remyelination. *Adv Exp Med Biol* 1999; **468**: 183–97.
11. Halliday AM, McDonald WI, Mushin J. Visual evoked response in diagnosis of multiple sclerosis. *Br Med J* 1973; **4**: 661–4.
12. Asselman P, Chadwick DW, Marsden CD. Visual evoked responses in the diagnosis and management of patients suspected of multiple sclerosis. *Brain* 1975; **98**: 261–82.
13. Gronseth GS, Ashman EJ. Practice parameter: The usefulness of evoked potentials in identifying clinically silent lesions in patients with suspected multiple sclerosis (an evidence-based review): Report of the Quality Standards Subcommittee of the American Academy of Neurology. *Neurology* 2000; **54**: 1720–5.
14. Odom JV, Bach M, Brigell M, Holder GE, McCulloch DL, Tormene AP. ISCEV standard for clinical visual evoked potentials (2009 update). *Doc Ophthalmol* 2010; **120**: 111–19.
15. Confavreux C, Vukusic S, Moreau T, Adeleine P. Relapses and progression of disability in multiple sclerosis. *N Engl J Med* 2000; **343**: 1430–8.
16. Bronnum-Hansen H, Koch-Henriksen N, Hyllested K. Survival of patients with multiple sclerosis in Denmark: a nationwide long-term epidemiologic survey. *Neurology* 1994; **44**: 1901–7.
17. Weinshenker BG, Bass B, Rice GPA. The natural history of multiple sclerosis: a geographically based study. 1. Clinical course and disability. *Brain* 1989; **112**: 133–46.
18. Arnold AC. Evolving management of optic neuritis and multiple sclerosis. *Am J Ophthalmol* 2005; **139**: 1101–8.
19. Rodriguez M, Siva A, Cross SA, O'Brien PC, Kurland LT. Optic neuritis: a population-based study in Olmsted County, Minnesota. *Neurology* 1995; **45**: 244–50.
20. Holder GE. The incidence of abnormal pattern electroretinography in optic nerve demyelination. *Electroenceph Clin Neurophysiol* 1991; **78**: 18–26.
21. Walsh JC, Garrick R, Cameron J, McLeod JG. Evoked potential changes in clinically definite multiple sclerosis: a two year follow-up study. *J Neurol Neurosurg Psychiatry* 1982; **45**: 494–500.
22. Frederiksen JL, Petrera J. Serial visual evoked potentials in 90 untreated patients with acute optic neuritis. *Surv Ophthalmol* 1999; **44**(S1): S54–62.
23. Hely MA, McManis PG, Walsh JC, McLeod JG. Visual evoked responses and ophthalmological examination in optic neuritis. A follow-up study. *J Neurol Sci* 1986; **75**: 275–83.
24. Matthews WB, Small M. Prolonged follow-up of abnormal visual evoked potentials in multiple sclerosis: evidence for delayed recovery. *J Neurol Neurosurg Psychiatry* 1983; **46**: 639–43.
25. Cusick JF, Myklebust JB, Larson SJ, Sances A. Spinal cord evaluation by cortical evoked responses. *Arch Neurol* 1979; **36**: 140–3.
26. Giblin DR. Somatosensory evoked potentials in healthy subjects and in patients with lesions of the nervous system. *Ann NY Acad Sci* 1964; **112**: 93–142.
27. Aminoff MJ, Eisen AA. Somatosensory evoked potentials. *Muscle Nerve* 1998; **21**: 277–90.
28. Aminoff MJ. The use of somatosensory evoked potentials in the evaluation of the central nervous system. *Neurol Clin* 1988; **6**: 809–23.
29. Cruccu G, Aminoff MJ, Curio G, et al. Recommendations for the clinical use of somatosensory-evoked potentials. *Clin Neurophysiol* 2008; **119**: 1705–19.
30. Chen R, Cros D, Curra A, et al. The clinical diagnostic utility of transcranial magnetic stimulation: Report of an IFCN committee. *Clin Neurophysiol* 2008; **119**: 504–32.
31. Webber M, Eisen AA. Magnetic stimulation of the central and peripheral nervous systems. *Muscle Nerve* 2002; **25**: 160–75.
32. Chiappa KH. *Evoked Potentials in Clinical Medicine*, 3rd edn. Philadelphia: Lippincott-Raven, 1997.
33. Purves SJ, Low MD, Galloway J, Reeves B. A comparison of visual, brainstem auditory and somatosensory evoked potentials in multiple sclerosis. *Can J Neurol Sci* 1981; **8**: 15–19.
34. Chiappa KH. Pattern shift visual, brainstem auditory, and short-latency somatosensory evoked potentials in multiple sclerosis. *Neurology* 1980; **30**: 110–23.

Chapter 5

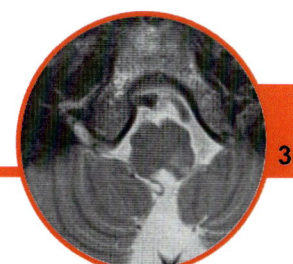

Multiple sclerosis differential diagnosis and mimics

Giles Elrington

The diagnosis of MS is essentially clinical; in other words, the diagnosis relies on the patient's symptoms and neurological examination, ideally while symptomatic. It is also most commonly a retrospective diagnosis, which brings dissatisfaction, as the diagnosis may seem obvious with hindsight. Worse than the diagnosis of MS, however, is an erroneous diagnosis of MS.

The differential diagnoses of MS relapse and of MS progression are very different.

Diagnostic criteria change with time, but the fundamentals remain constant. The diagnosis of RRMS relies upon 'dissemination in time and place' i.e. lesions at different times in different parts of the CNS.

Acute relapses of existing RRMS present scaled-down challenges similar to the diagnosis of MS itself; however, to be newly diagnosed with MS requires a higher level of proof than diagnosing a new relapse in established RRMS. It is a common mistake to assume that all neurological symptoms in a person with RRMS must be caused by MS relapse.

Progressive MS is a more challenging diagnosis but essentially requires evidence of both inflammation and degeneration (i.e. deterioration over time). In SPMS, the previous relapses give evidence of inflammation; in PPMS (the most difficult type to diagnose) CSF analysis proves inflammation.

In principle, RRMS can be diagnosed entirely on clinical grounds with no investigations, though that is now unusual. Investigation is mandatory to diagnose progressive forms of MS. These investigations may strengthen or weaken a clinical diagnosis of MS.

The definition of MS is inclusive, not exclusive: either the diagnostic criteria are fulfilled (patient has MS) or they are not (MS cannot be diagnosed in this patient today). There are no specific diagnostic criteria for 'not having MS', though the following may be inferred:

1. A symptomatic patient who has a normal CNS examination does not have symptoms of MS.
2. A person with a normal MRI scan of the entire CNS, and normal CSF examination [no oligoclonal bands (OCBs) unique to the CSF] does not have MS.

These statements assume that normality of examination and MRI are easily defined: they are not.

Dual pathology presents particular problems to the diagnosis of MS and MS relapse.

Diagnosis in MS eventually comes down to a matter of pattern recognition for the experienced specialist. Non-specialists tend to rely more on investigations; it is easy to see MS in terms of symptoms and MRI scans, often with CSF data. This overlooks the critical importance of the neurological examination, which must be abnormal at some point in a patient with MS.

The fundamental difficulty is that there is no 'gold standard' or 'bottom-line' test for MS; everything that can be abnormal in MS, from physical examination to MRI and CSF, can be found in other conditions. Putting together the whole picture of the diagnosis is like assembling a jigsaw in which no one piece gives the full picture.

It is all too easy, erroneously, to assume that any of the following equate to a diagnosis of MS:

1. MRI reported as showing MS;
2. positive CSF OCBs;
3. on treatment for MS;
4. seeing the MS nurse;
5. member of MS patient support group.

Multiple sclerosis relapse

Most people with MS (85%) begin the illness with attacks, relapses or episodes. These are usually young adults aged 20–40, though no age group is exempt.

By definition, relapses last at least 24 hours. In practice, they normally last weeks or months; onset is normally over hours or days, not abrupt or maximal at onset. Symptoms usually remain static and then improve gradually. There is no maximum relapse duration: in some clinical trials, persistent worsening lasting 3 months has been assumed to equate to progression, whereas in routine clinical practice the threshold of a year is sometimes used. The only time that relapse can be distinguished from progression with compete certainty, is at recovery.

Average relapse frequency is once or twice a year, although there is a very wide range. Relapse frequency tends to diminish over time.

MS symptoms can be mimicked by increased body heat while pyrexial with an infection, or from exercise or ambient temperature. This is termed a pseudo-relapse, though it is a very real problem. Reprise of former symptoms in the setting of pyrexia or other evidence of active infection, is not considered a true relapse for the purposes of diagnosis or treatment decision.

MS relapses typically affect the optic nerve (painful monocular visual loss), brainstem (double vision, clumsiness, paralysis) or spinal cord (paralysis, sensory loss, bladder difficulty). Sequential bilateral optic neuritis does not give dissemination in time and place, thus MS, as there is a broad differential diagnosis, including chiasmal (pituitary) disease, Leber's optic neuropathy, and other inflammatory optic neuritides, including sarcoidosis and neuromyelitis optica (Devic's disease; **5.1**).

MS relapse, with symptoms usually maturing over hours or days, may, surprisingly, be mimicked by other acute or episodic neurological attacks, including cerebrovascular disease (transient ischaemic attack and stroke; **5.2, 5.3**) in which symptoms are maximal at onset; and migraine aura in which symptoms mature over a matter of minutes.

5.1 (A) Longitudinally extensive spinal cord lesion seen on T2-weighted MRI in neuromyelitis optica (Devic's disease). The cord appears grossly swollen, with the lesion extending from the high cervical spinal cord to the thoracic cord. (B) It can be seen that the lesion is central within the spinal cord on axial MRI.

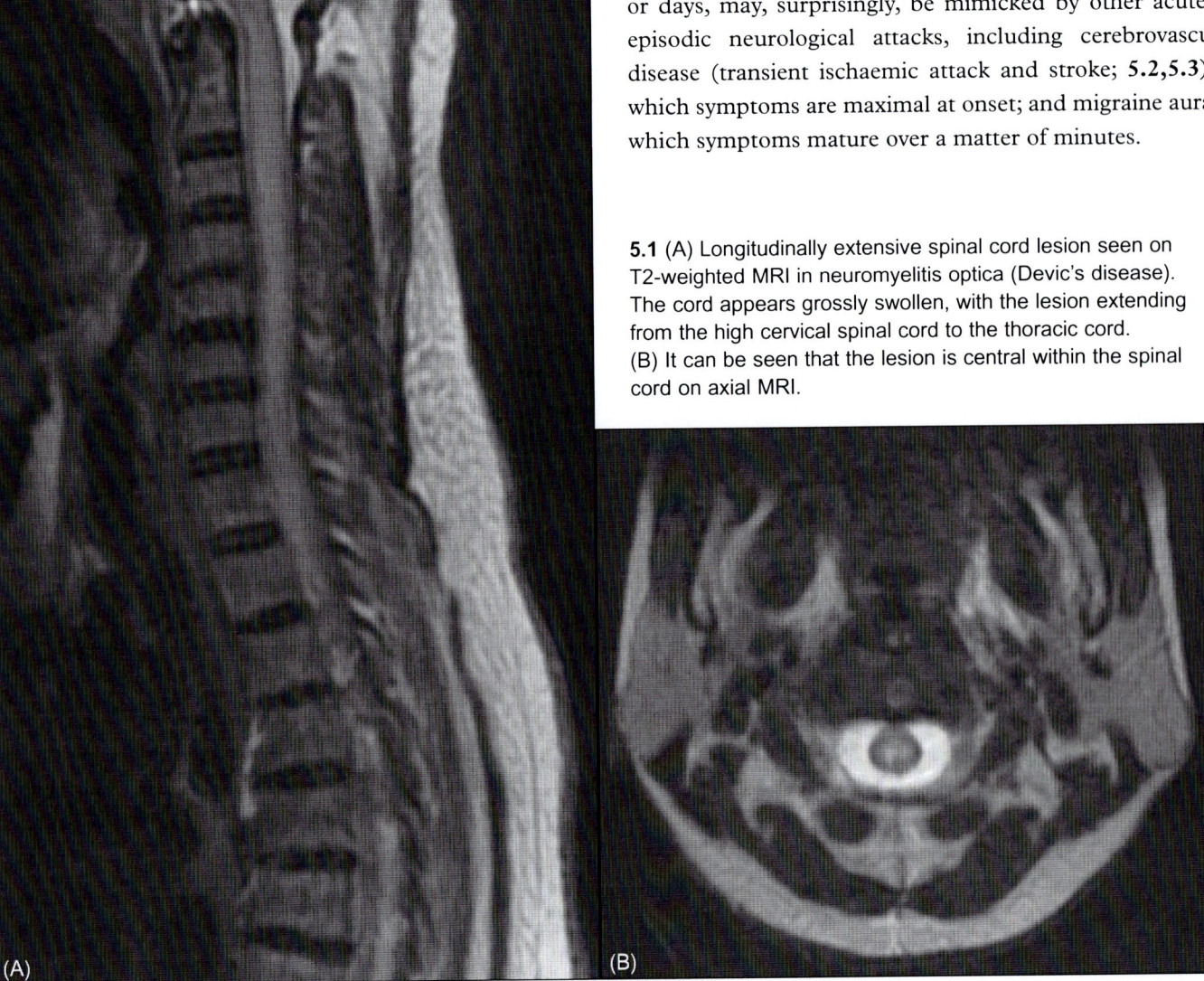

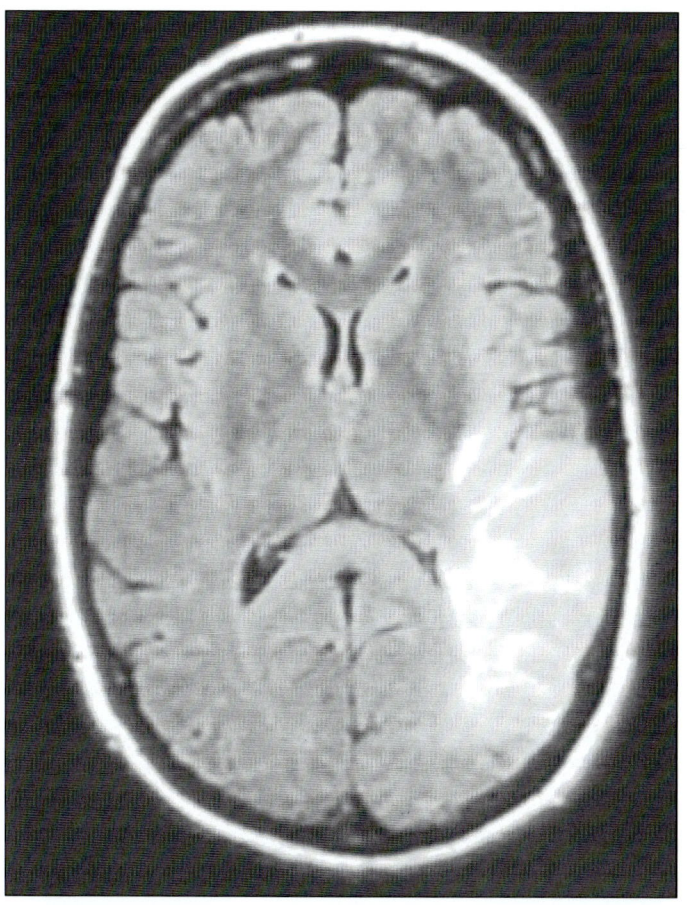

Multiple sclerosis differential diagnosis and mimics 33

5.2 Acute left middle cerebral artery stroke. The abrupt onset of symptoms in this patient indicated a vascular origin, and would not usually be confused with MS, in contrast to small vessel vascular disease (see **5.7**).

5.3 Acute brainstem infarction shown on T2-weighted MRI (A) and diffusion-weighted images (DWI) (B,C). This patient presented with acute onset vertigo, hiccoughs and vomiting. On examination, there was left-sided ataxia with right-sided sensory disturbance. While the brainstem is a typical site for MS plaques, the restriction on the DWI (B) confirms the vascular cause of his symptoms. The first DWI image shows a 'bright' (*white*) lesion (B, *arrowed*), indicating abnormal water diffusion in that area. The second image, the apparent diffusion coefficient map, shows a dark (*black*) lesion (C, *arrowed*), confirming the ischaemic nature of the lesion.

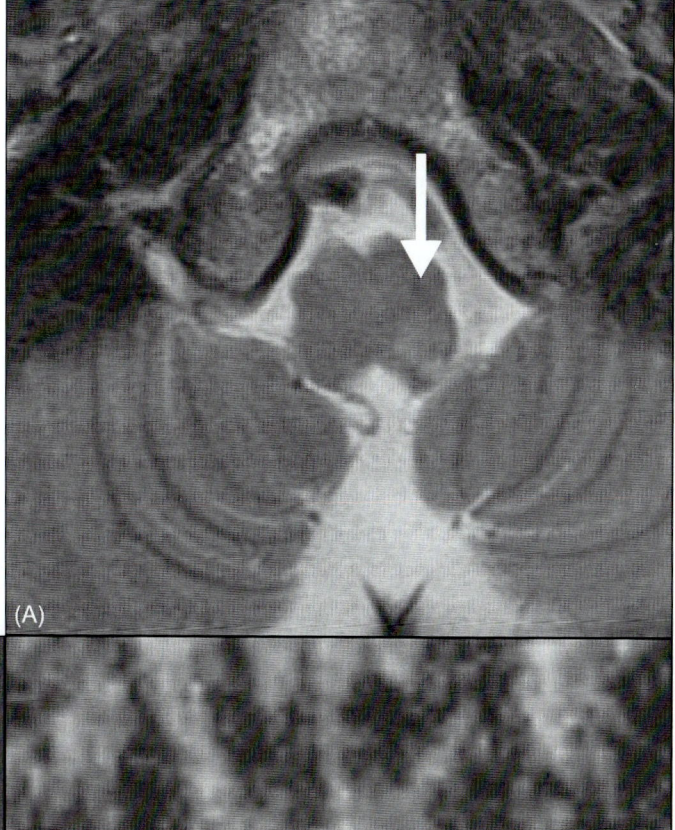

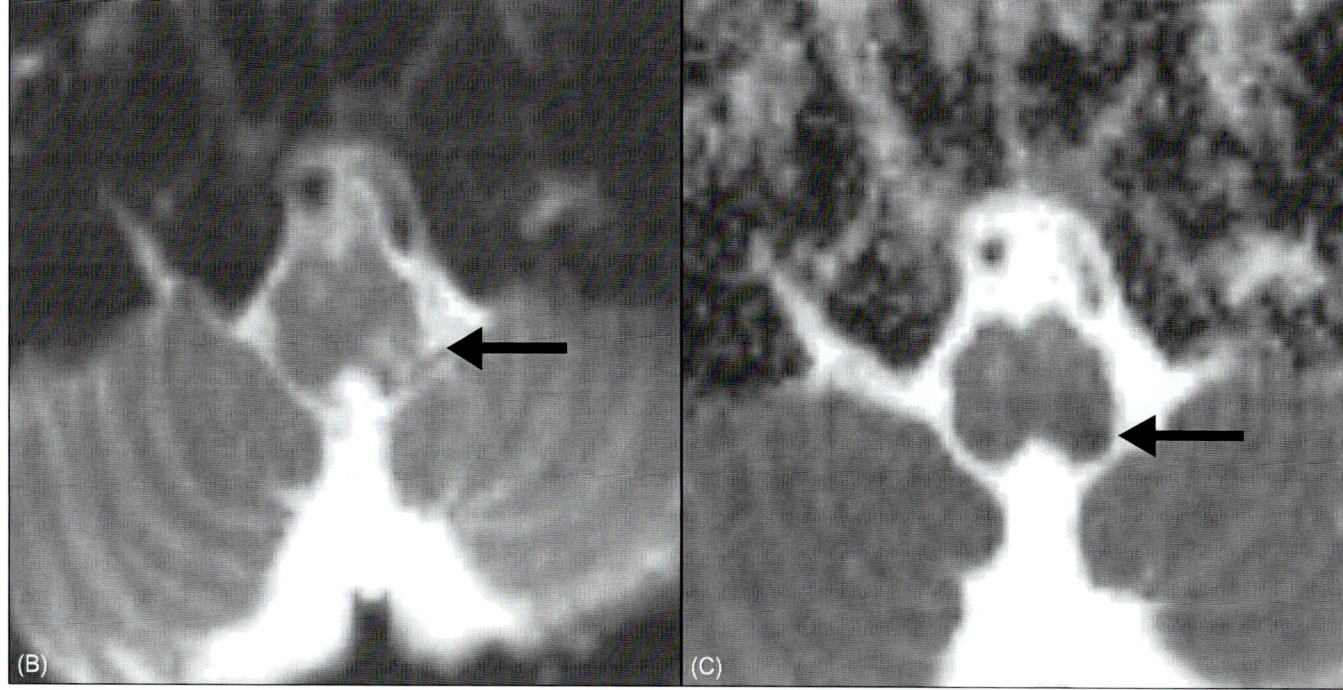

34 Multiple sclerosis differential diagnosis and mimics

Other systemic autoimmune conditions can mimic RRMS, including lupus in its many forms, which can be suspected from anticardiolipin and other immunological blood tests, and sarcoidosis (**5.4**), an immune disorder of uncertain cause. These typically cause problems beyond the CNS, which in the setting of '?MS' may require further investigation. Acute disseminated encephalomyelitis (**5.5**) is a monophasic CNS disorder usually seen in children following viral infection in which the MRI can look very like that of MS; 'relapse of acute disseminated encephalomyelitis' is usually RRMS.

Multiple sclerosis progression

SPMS is, with hindsight, normally a straightforward clinical diagnosis, but it is very difficult to know exactly when the patient moves from RRMS to SPMS. Otherwise, the key differential diagnosis is between other causes of progressive myelopathy, particularly cervical (rarely dorsal) spine compression by disc prolapse (**5.6**) or other mass lesions, including tumour and cyst (syringomyelia), and vitamin B12 deficiency.

PPMS is inevitably the most difficult form of MS to diagnose as it must be distinguished from the many other slowly progressive neurological disorders (**5.7**). There is a particular problem with possible multiple diagnosis: when a patient with RRMS gets gradually worse, how secure is the assumption of SPMS, or do other causes of progressive disease need to be excluded? Typically, this means investigation of the spinal cord; before MRI was widely available (in the UK this means the twentieth century) an invasive test, the myelogram, was needed, which is much more unpleasant than a lumbar puncture. It was not uncommon for people with progressive MS to blame the myelogram for their later decline. MS clinics still contain patients with progressive MS whose spinal cords have not been imaged; it is always hard to decide whether, late in the illness, a return to investigation is indicated.

Other neurodegenerative diseases may mimic progressive MS; some, like MS, cluster within families, such as the many types of hereditary spastic paraparesis in which CSF OCBs are not found. A particular trap for the investigation-reliant doctor is tropical spastic paraparesis in which CSF OCBs are found.

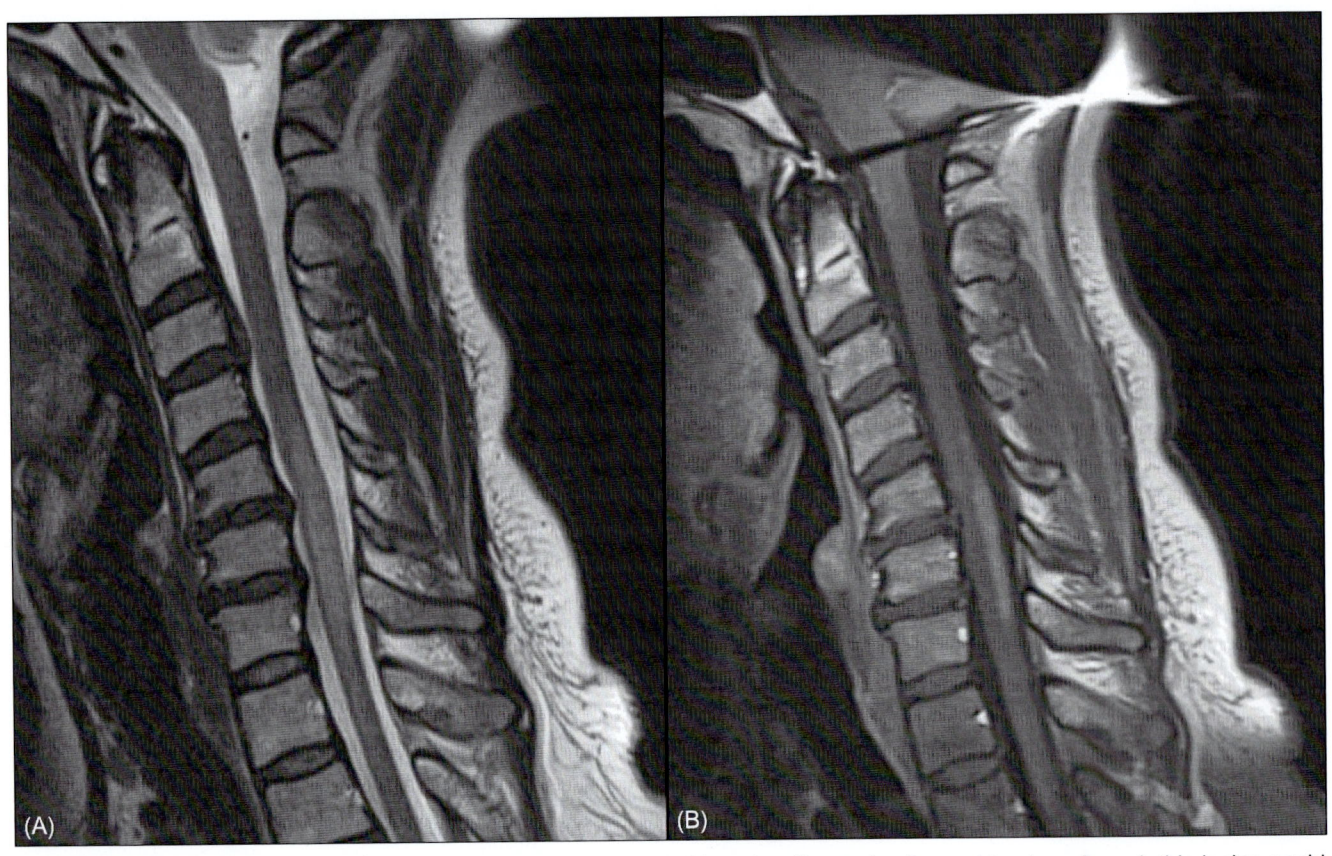

5.4 Cervical spine lesion in a patient with biopsy-proven sarcoid. Were the diagnosis of sarcoid not confirmed, this lesion could be in keeping with neuromyelitis optica, highlighting the relative non-specificity of MRI. (A) T2-weighted MRI. (B) T1-weighted MRI demonstrating gadolinium enhancement of the lesion.

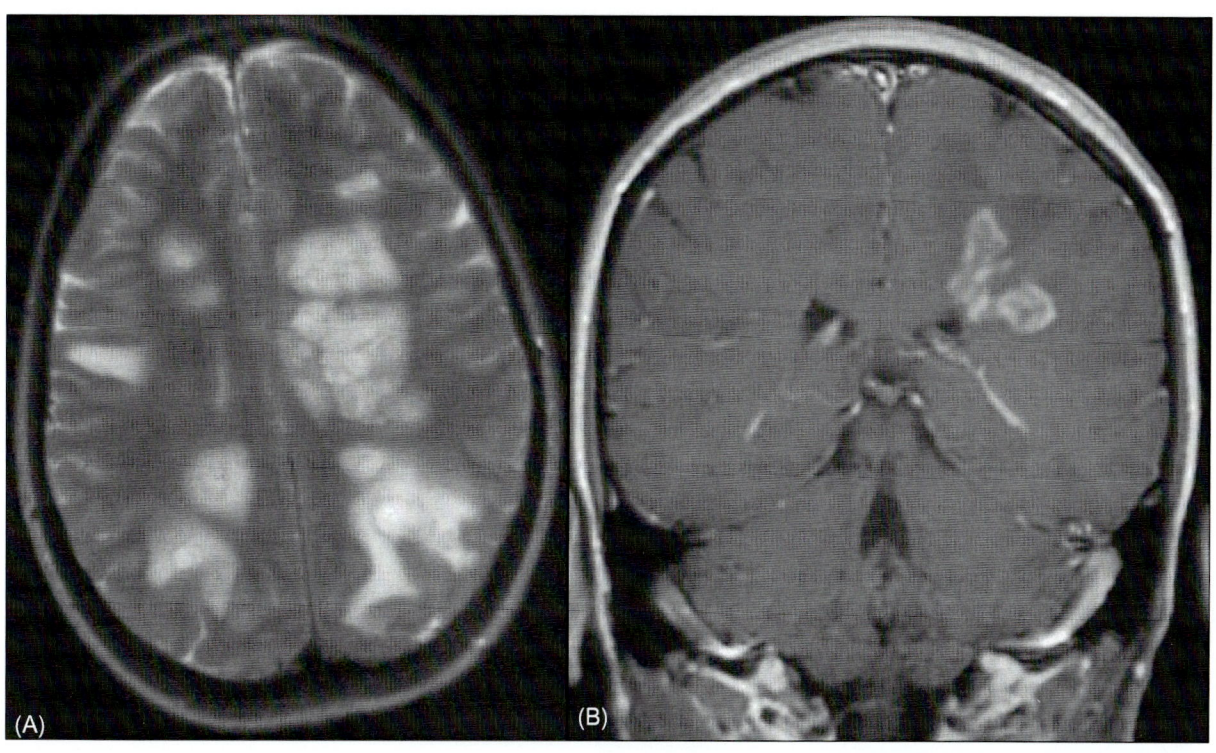

Multiple sclerosis differential diagnosis and mimics

5.5 (A) T2-weighted MRI appearances of a patient with acute disseminated encephalomyelitis (ADEM); however, it must be noted that there are many potential appearances of ADEM, a discussion of which is beyond the remit of this chapter. (B) T1 gadolinium-enhanced images of a patient with ADEM, demonstrating the florid enhancement that can be seen in patients with this condition.

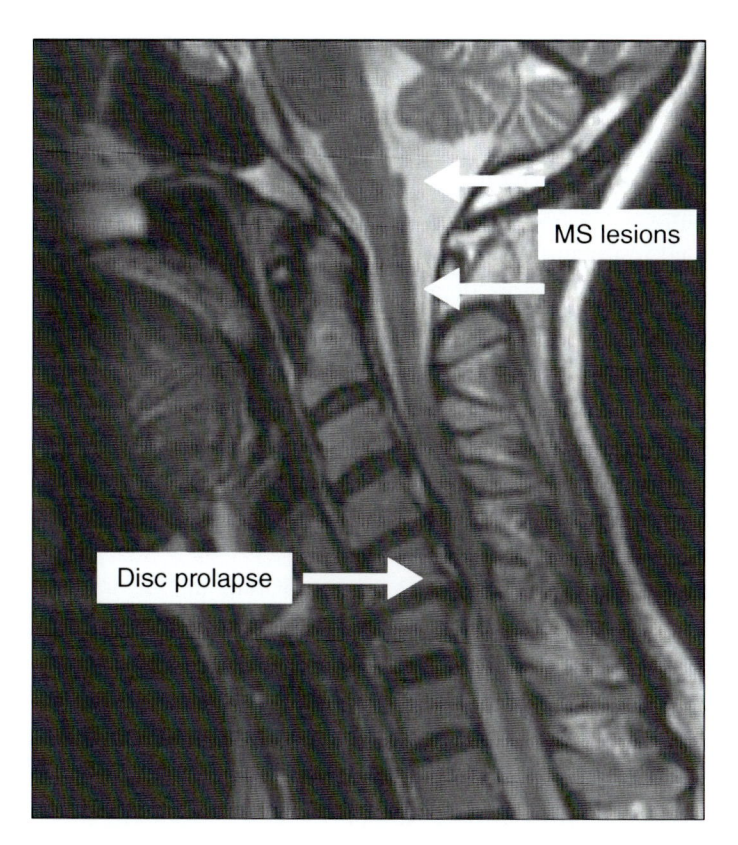

5.6 This patient was given a diagnosis of RRMS a few years earlier but later experienced progressive gait decline over several months. Examination revealed a spastic paraparesis. MRI cervical spine shows both the changes of MS in her spinal cord and brainstem; and cervical cord compression from cervical disc prolapse. Following technically successful decompresssive surgery her slow decline continued unabated and was eventually attributed to SPMS.

36 Multiple sclerosis differential diagnosis and mimics

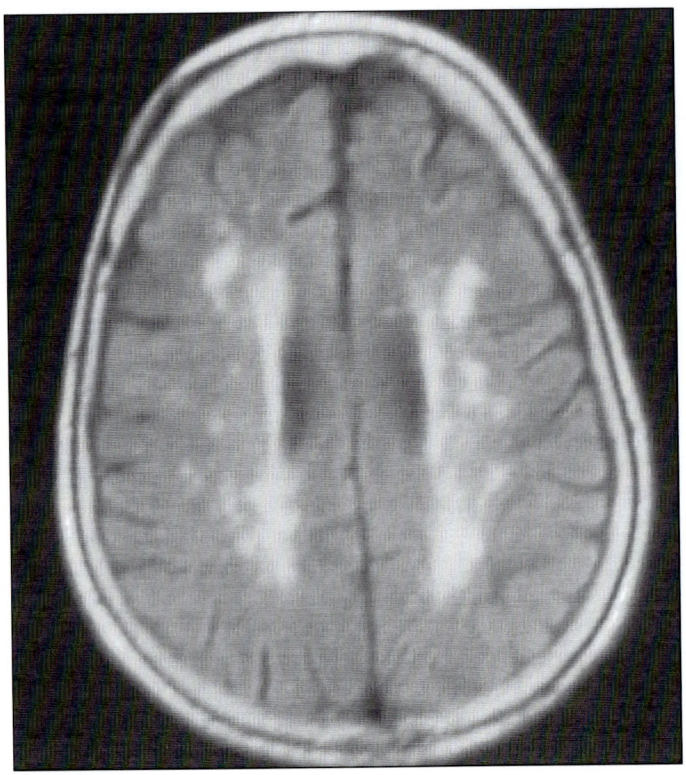

5.7 Small vessel cerebrovascular disease; this can give rise to a clinical picture mimicking progressive MS.

Specific multiple sclerosis mimics

In the specialist neurology clinic, a broad and esoteric differential may be considered. In 'real life', the first, and often overlooked consideration is 'something or nothing serious'. It is all too easy to interpret symptoms such as sensory loss, weakness, clumsiness, dizziness, visual difficulty, bowel, bladder and sexual dysfunction, and fatigue, as symptoms of MS. They are also symptoms of many other diseases and are often the presenting problem in people who achieve no neurological diagnosis.

Medically unexplained symptoms (MUS) account for about a third of new patients in the neurology clinic.[1] In the twentieth century this was known as somatization, implying the physical manifestation of covert psychosocial distress. Undoubtedly there is a psychiatric differential diagnosis, including a mood and personality disorder, but not everybody with MUS has a psychiatric problem and the newer term offers the great advantage of keeping an open mind. Many people with MUS are seriously disabled. A common subgroup of MUS is the chronic fatigue syndrome, which is easily mistaken for MS. To further complicate matters, there are some people with undoubted MS who behave just like a person with MUS, including 'non-organic' patterns of weakness.

Migraine is a common disorder affecting 5% of women, most often young women, and includes aura, which typically affects both eyes, and sensory change, weakness, tremor, speech difficulty and fatigue. Most migraine aura lasts an hour or less, but prolonged and atypical auras are also recognized, as is aura without headache, which affects 1–2% of the healthy population. A patient who died of treatment complications in an MS trial proved with autopsy and hindsight to have not MS, but migraine.[2]

Tests for multiple sclerosis

There is no 'gold standard' test for MS. Autopsy is generally reliable; brain biopsies are very rarely undertaken to distinguish 'tumefactive MS' from tumours such as lymphoma or metastasis, and from infections such as tuberculosis.

MRI scans are the most commonly used tests. The MRI brain scan shows lesions in 95% of people with RRMS, which is therefore not excluded by a normal MRI brain scan alone. The lesions of MS are notoriously non-specific being easily confused with 'unidentified bright objects', which normal people acquire at a rate of about one per decade, more in those with cerebrovascular risk factors, migraine aura and head injury. Normal spaces around blood vessels are also easily mistaken for MS lesions. The presence of gadolinium-enhancing lesion(s) greatly strengthens MRI support for MS where clinically appropriate; MRI is now used to demonstrate dissemination in time and place. MRI is discussed in more detail in Chapter 3.

Spinal MRI is less sensitive but more specific for MS than brain MRI; arguably the more important use of spinal MRI is to exclude alternative and surgically treatable causes of myelopathy (spinal cord disease).

The big problem with MRI is its non-specificity and particularly the high chance of incidental findings. One in four healthy teenagers has disc prolapse on spinal MRI; brain MRI is 'not strictly normal' in one in four healthy 20-year-olds and 1 in 40 healthy adults has a significant abnormality.[3]

CSF analysis may be more useful to exclude than to confirm MS. The key test is for OCBs of immunoglobulin unique to the CSF. Modern analysis techniques have improved the sensitivity of OCB testing; the finding of no excess OCBs

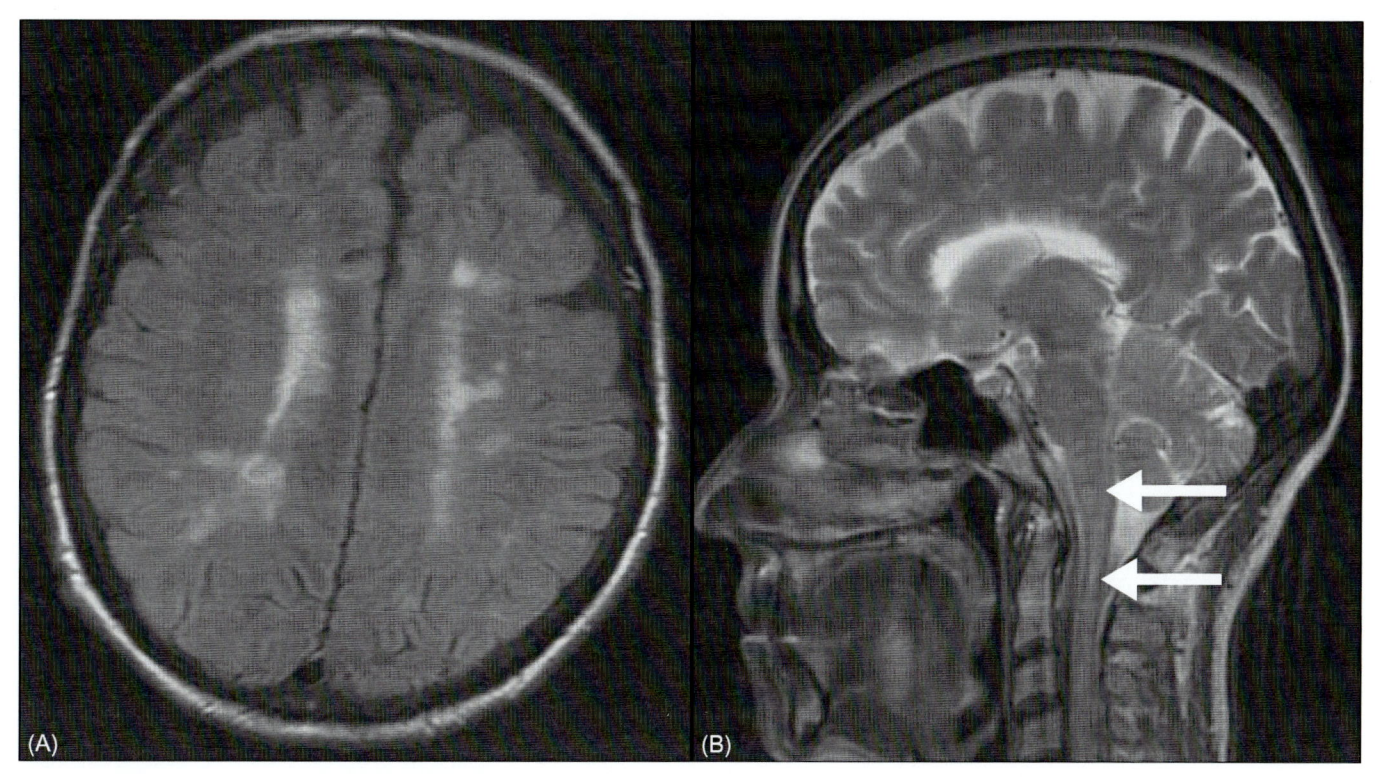

5.8 MS mistaken for cerebrovascular disease. This patient had a number of neurological episodes initially thought to be transient ischaemic attacks. The MRI brain scan was reported to show cerebrovascular disease. A cardiac cause (patent foramen ovale) was diagnosed and repaired, but her attacks continued. A further MRI a few months later at a different hospital was reported by the same general radiologist as showing MS. Neurological review found no interval change on the MRI but it was felt that the brainstem and cervical spine changes in particular were more suggestive of MS than cerebrovascular disease. CSF contained oligoclonal bands. The possibility that she has both MS and cerebrovascular disease cannot be excluded. (A) Axial T2 FLAIR MRI. (B) Sagittal T2 MRI showing brainstem and cervical spinal cord lesions (*arrowed*).

in CSF either excludes, or casts very substantial doubt on, a diagnosis of MS. CSF OCBs are found in a small minority of healthy people, so this finding alone does not prove MS. Absence of a contemporaneous blood sample invalidates the CSF analysis. In addition, the finding of the same OCBs in CSF and blood is, for MS diagnostic purposes, effectively a negative result. Patients do not generally enjoy CSF being obtained at lumbar puncture, though in experienced hands the procedure does not justify its fearsome reputation.

Electrical tests of CNS conduction, evoked potentials, can be used to provide evidence of dissemination in place (see Chapter 4 for more details on these). Thus, a patient with myelopathy and delayed VEPs probably has MS. VEPs do not, however, contribute to current diagnostic criteria, having been largely superseded by MRI. The VEP can occasionally be helpful as a negative; if normal, monocular visual impairment is unlikely to be MS related.

Blood tests are generally uninformative in MS; however, they will sometimes suggest alternative diagnoses such as thyroid disease, lupus, vitamin B12 deficiency, or neuromyelitis optica, which in many but not all cases associates with anti-aquaporin-4 antibodies.

Conclusions

The differential diagnosis of MS ranges from the mundane to the esoteric. A diagnosis of MS is always fundamentally clinical and needs critical re-analysis over time. No test is perfect in confirming MS.

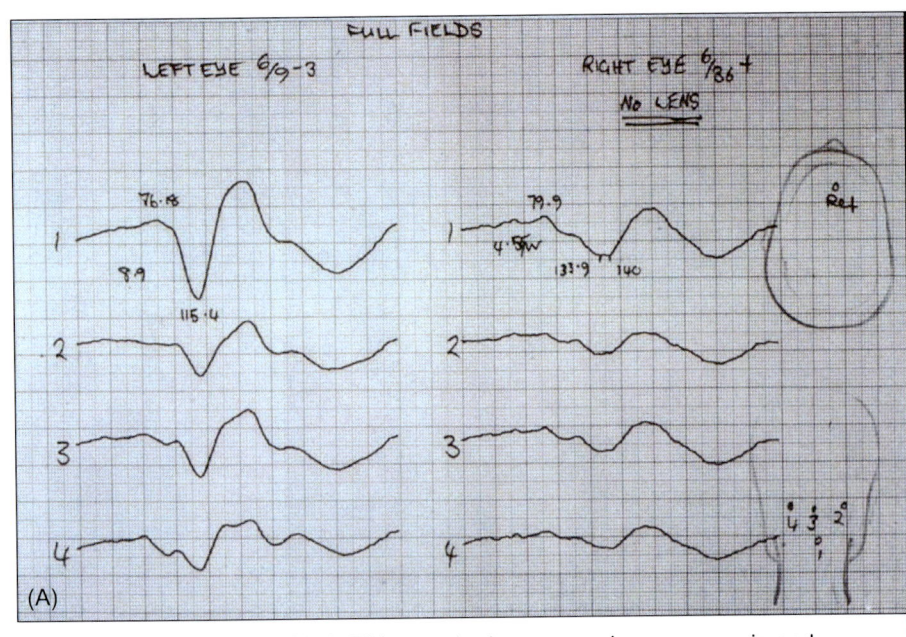

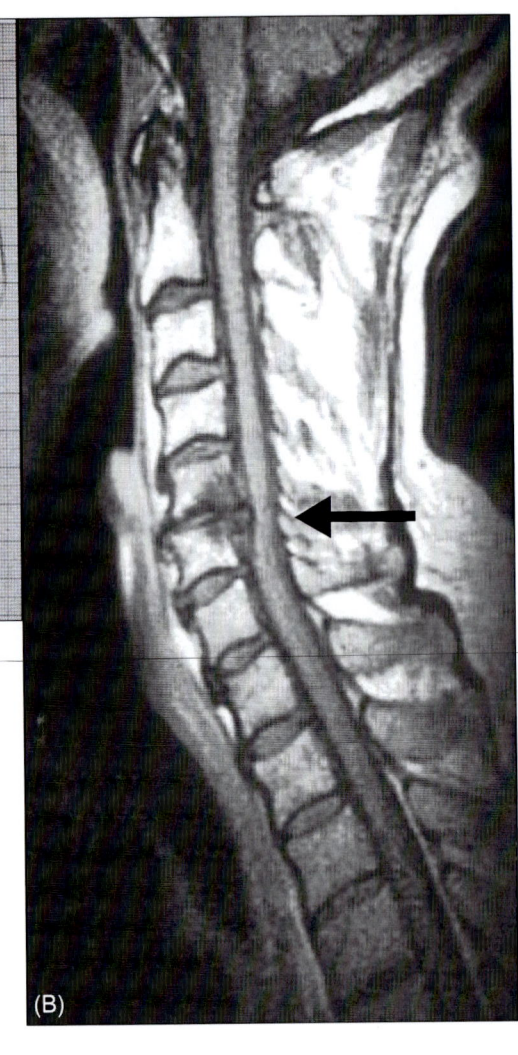

38 Multiple sclerosis differential diagnosis and mimics

5.9 Erroneous diagnosis of MS. This man had a progressive paraparesis and was given a diagnosis of MS by a general physician in the 1980s based upon abnormal visual evoked potentials (A). In fact, the abnormality is explained by old trauma to the eye; at neurological review in the early 1990s the diagnosis was re-evaluated and MRI of the cervical spine showed cervical spinal cord compression by disc prolapse (B, *arrowed*), which was surgically treated, halting but not reversing his previous progression.

References

1. Carson AJ, Ringbauer B, Stone J, et al. Do medically unexplained symptoms matter? A prospective cohort study of 300 new referrals to neurology outpatient clinic. *J Neurol Neurosurg Psychiatry* 2000; **68**: 207–10.
2. Chaudhari A. Lessons for clinical trials from Natalizumab in multiple sclerosis. *Br Med J* 2006; **332**: 416.
3. Morris Z, Whiteley W, Longstreth WT, et al. Incidental findings no brain magnetic resonance imaging: systematic review and meta-analysis. *Br Med J* 2009; **339**: 547–50.

Chapter 6

Pathology of multiple sclerosis
Part 1 – Human

Sandra Amor and Paul van der Valk

History of MS pathology

The French neurologist Jean-Martin Charcot (1825–1893) (**6.1**) is generally credited with the first full description of the neuropathology of MS as well as recognizing that MS was a distinct clinical entity.[1] His intense interest in the pathology together with his findings in MS led to the disease initially being known as Charcot's disease. Jean Charcot originally called the disease *la sclerose en plaques disseminées*, and only later did it become known as MS after the German terminology *multiple Sklerose*.

Gross pathology

While all regions of the CNS may be affected, lesions occur in predilection sites such as the optic nerves, chiasm and brain stem. In severe chronic cases, atrophy of the brain and spinal cord is observed. Dissection of the brain post mortem reveals greyish shrunken lesions in the white matter (**6.2**) that are often firm to the touch due to fibrous scar tissue formation. Such lesions are frequently associated with blood vessels, and where lesions spread along large vessels they are called Dawson's fingers after the Scottish pathologist James Walker Dawson (1870–1927). As well as white matter lesions, more detailed examination of the brain also reveals lesions within the cortical regions referred to as grey matter lesions.

White matter lesions

The areas in the white matter that do not contain classically demyelinated lesions frequently reveal subtle abnormalities when examined microscopically and using imaging studies.[2,3] As the myelin appears normal in routine myelin stains these areas are called 'normal-appearing white matter' (**6.3**). Thus, while gross pathology shows little change in the white matter, imaging and microscopy reveal ongoing tissue damage and repair mechanisms.

6.1 Jean-Martin Charcot was born in Paris, France, in 1825 and died in 1893. Charcot was the founder of modern neurology and described the pathology of MS once referred to as Charcot's disease.

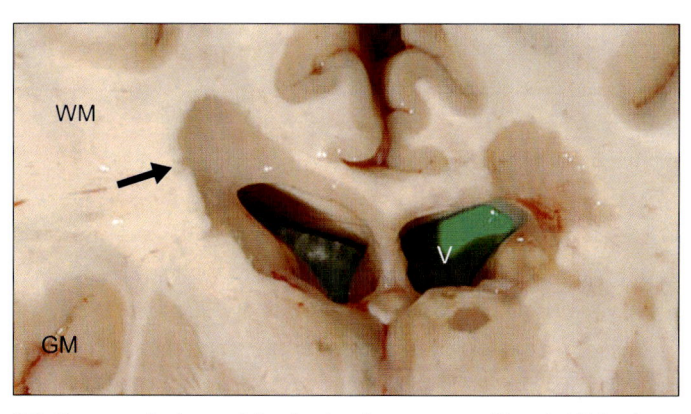

6.2 Gross pathology of the brain of a person with established MS shows the typical scar lesions (*arrow*) surrounding the ventricles (V). GM, cortical grey matter (the green area is the supporting cloth); WM, white matter.

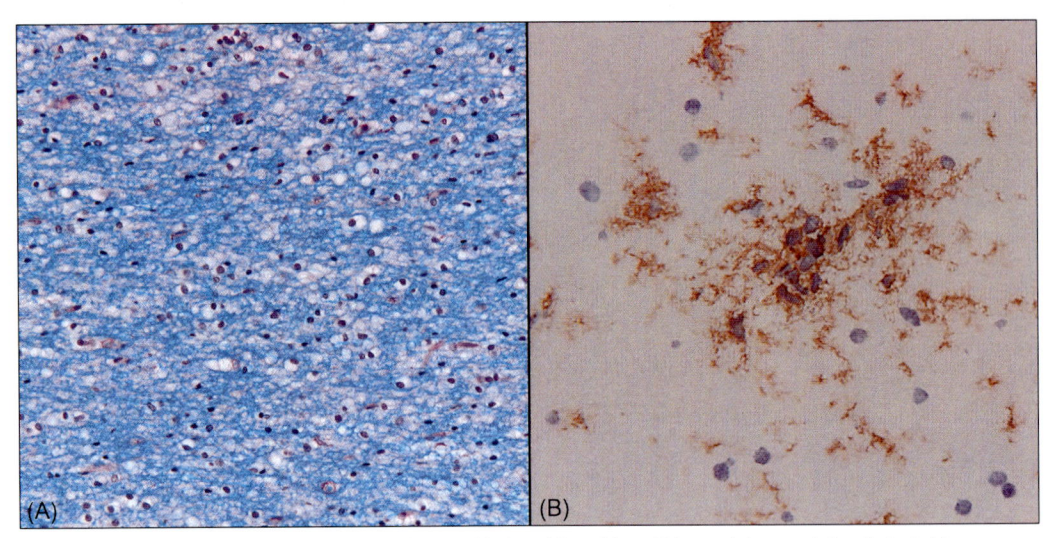

6.3 Normal-appearing white matter stained with luxol fast blue (A), nuclei are stained dark blue. (B) In normal-appearing white matter a cluster of activated microglia depicted by immunohistochemical staining for major histocompatibility complex II (*brown*) form a preactive MS lesion.

In some cases, large areas of diffusely (or 'dirty') abnormal white matter are observed by imaging studies. These areas correlate with less intense myelin staining, an increase in astrocyte activity and depletion of axons.

Preactive lesions

Preactive lesions are characterized by discrete clusters of activated microglia in areas of otherwise normal-appearing myelin (**6.3**). These lesions are not associated with blood vessels or other lesions, indicating that they may be triggered by stressed oligodendrocytes (the myelin forming cells).[4] That the preactive lesions outnumber all other white matter lesions suggests that in most cases activation of microglia and thus these lesions resolve with time. The rare finding of Oil-red O-positive material within phagocytic cells reflecting transition to an active lesion suggests why some preactive lesions develop into active lesions.

Active lesions

The presence of a solid mass of lipid-laden (Oil-red-O) foamy macrophages (**6.4A**) that highly express the immune molecular major histocompatibility complex II (**6.4B**) is characteristic of active MS lesions.[5] The stage or age of the lesion is reflected by differential immunoreactivity of macrophage phagosomes for certain myelin proteins. At the last stage, only Oil-red-O-positive neutral lipids persist, while all myelin proteins have been fully degraded. Axonal bulbs and spheroids representing axonal damage are observed together with thickened axons very prominently in active MS lesions.[6] In these lesions oligodendrocytes show signs of stress due to the expression of heat shock proteins. Some active lesions contain increased numbers of oligodendrocytes, probably recruited from the precursor pool, while in other lesions oligodendrocyte numbers are decreased, clearly indicating cell death.[7] Blood vessels associated with perivascular cellular infiltrates (**6.4C**) are frequently observed within active lesions while astrocytes show signs of hypertrophy and express glial fibrillary acid protein referred to as 'reactive gliosis'.

Chronic active lesions

As myelin is degraded, the active lesion becomes depleted of myelin (**6.5**), and the phagocytic macrophages are only present at the lesion's rim leaving an hypocellular centre (**6.5A–C**) characteristic of the chronic active lesion. At the edge of some lesions, oligodendrocyte numbers are increased, probably reflecting remyelination that can even be observed in patents with long-standing disease. However, oligodendrocytes are severely depleted in the centre and astrocytes become reactive forming the gliotic scar.

Chronic inactive lesions

In time, the number of phagocytosing macrophages in the rim decreases, the activity dies out and the inactive lesion is formed (**6.6**). This is the typical grey, sunken, sclerotic lesion seen upon macroscopy. It is usually a completely demyelinated area (**6.6A**), and is hypocellular throughout (**6.6B**) with isomorphic gliosis and hypertrophic astrocytes (**6.6C**).

Pathology of multiple sclerosis part 1 – human

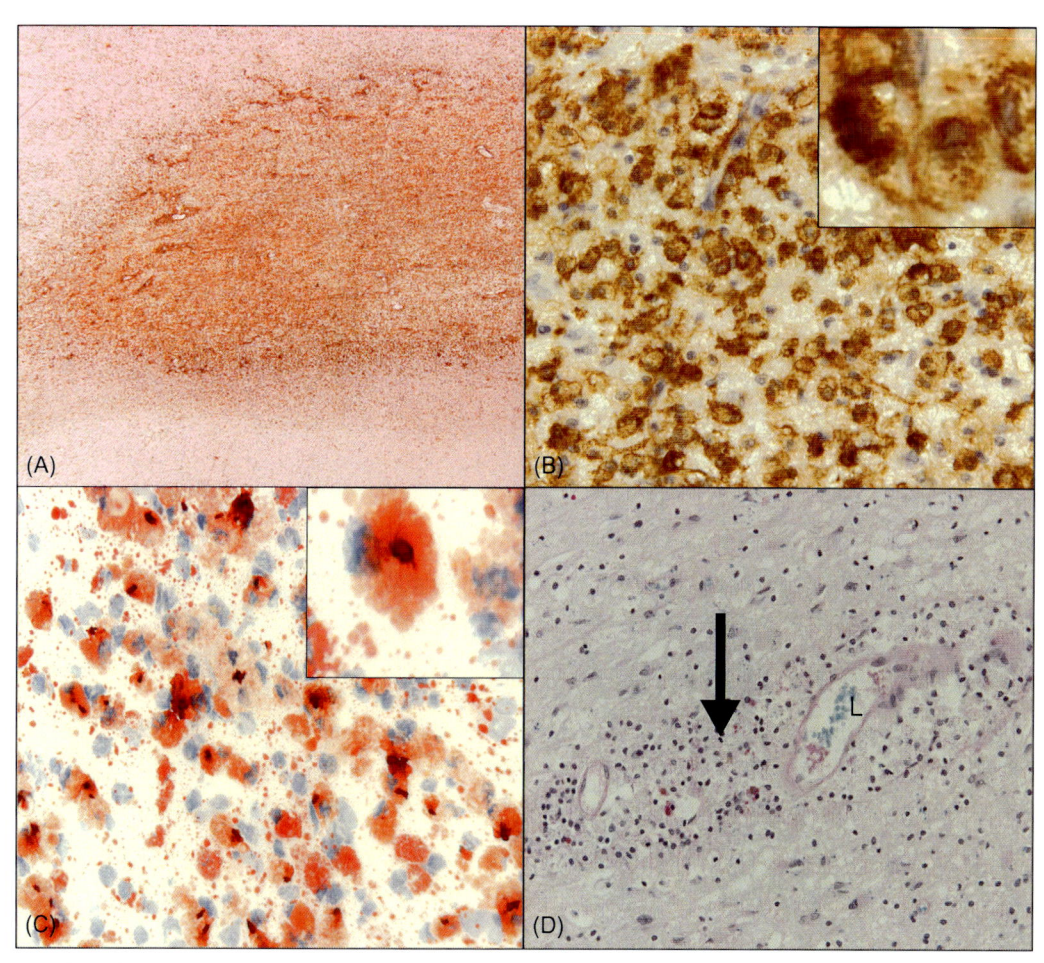

6.4 Active lesions contain activated major histocompatibility complex class II positive cells (A, overview; B, low power) that display the immune molecule major histocompatibility complex II. Inset: three highly activated phagocytes. These cells contain oil-red-O-positive neutral lipids (C) indicative of uptake of myelin by macrophages/microglia. Inset: lipid droplets inside a phagocytic cell. (D) Macrophages and lymphocytes (*arrow*) are present within the perivascular area of a blood vessel within or close to the active lesion. L, lumen of the blood vessel.

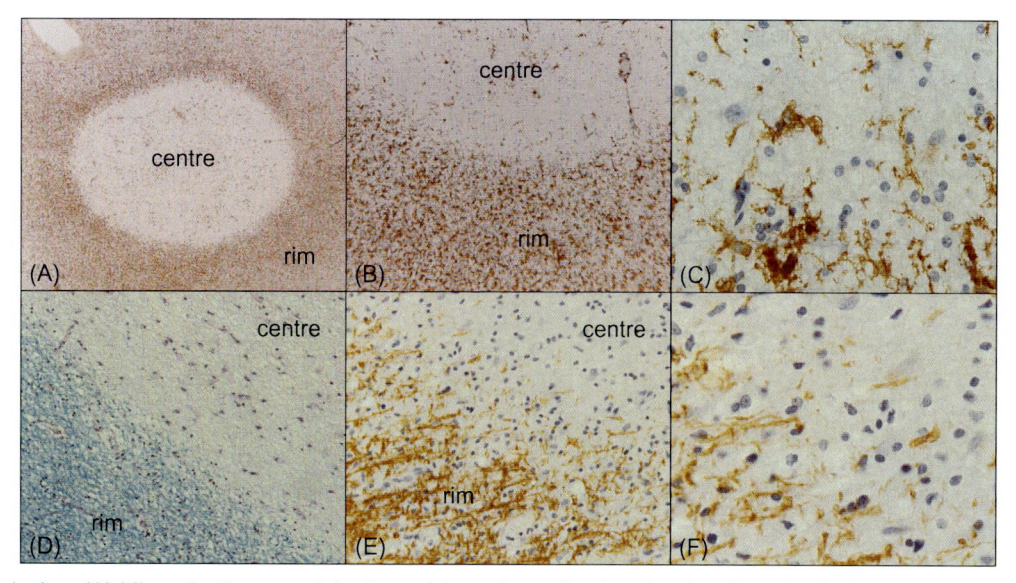

6.5 Chronic active lesion. (A) Microglia (immunostain, *brown*) have formed a rim of a chronic active lesion leaving a hypocellular centre. (B, C) High power showing that microglia are highly active. While the edge (rim) of the lesion contains myelin (*blue* in D, *brown* in E) the centre is completely demyelinated. A high-power picture shows wisps of myelin (F) brown at the inner edge of the rim of a chronic active lesion.

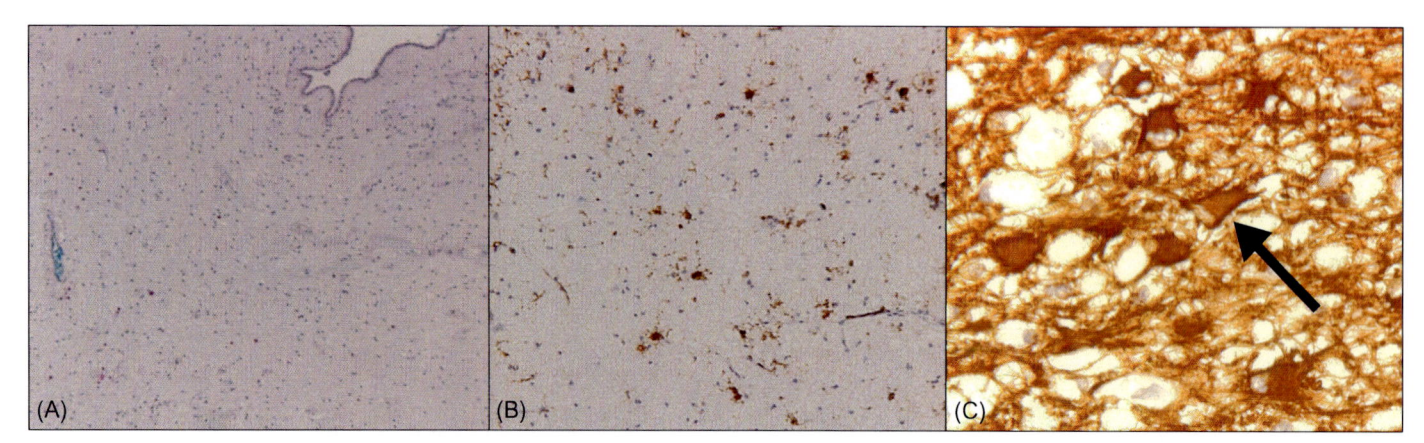

42 Pathology of multiple sclerosis part 1 – human

6.6 Inactive lesions are completed demyelinated (A, *luxol fast blue*) as seen in this periventricular lesion. The hypocellular centre is almost devoid of activated macrophages (B), yet is populated by hypertrophic astrocytes (C, *arrow*) forming gliotic scar (*stained brown*).

The size and numbers of acute, chronic active and inactive lesions vary with each case and lesions may coalesce. Examination of a large cohort of patients with MS has revealed that different lesions in the brain of one person often appear to be at a similar stage. In addition, some patients develop many grey matter lesions, while others develop predominantly white matter lesions. The different stages of lesions suggest a sequence of lesion formation beginning with the clusters of activated microglia in preactive lesions, followed by active and chronic active and finally the sclerotic inactive MS lesions. The degree of remyelination is very variable[8] and appears at the edge of chronic active lesions or as discreet areas in the brain called shadow plaques.

Grey matter pathology

Despite being recognized by Charcot, the detailed study of grey matter damage in MS was largely ignored until the last decade due to the lack of sophisticated detection methods. Similar to white matter lesions, myelin damage is observed in both the cortical as well as deep grey matter. However, in contrast, infiltration of B cells, T cells, and macrophages is largely absent from grey matter lesions, as is clear blood–brain barrier (BBB) damage.

Cortical pathology is classified on the basis of the anatomical localization of the lesion.[9] The *leucocorticoid lesion* (**6.7A**) is a combined grey and white matter lesion, in which myelin damage affects both brain regions. Interestingly, myelin loss is seen in both the white and grey matter regions while microglia activation is largely restricted to the white matter. Recent results from our group suggest that myelin debris released during demyelination is a major factor stimulating the inflammatory response.[10] The *intracortical lesion* (**6.7B**) is similar to the grey matter part of a leucocorticoid lesion. The subpial lesions (**6.7C**) are seen as 'ribbons' of demyelination directly below the leptomeninges and may be extensive covering the entire surface of the brain.

Myelin damage and loss is also seen in the deep grey matter, such as the thalamus and caudate, putamen,

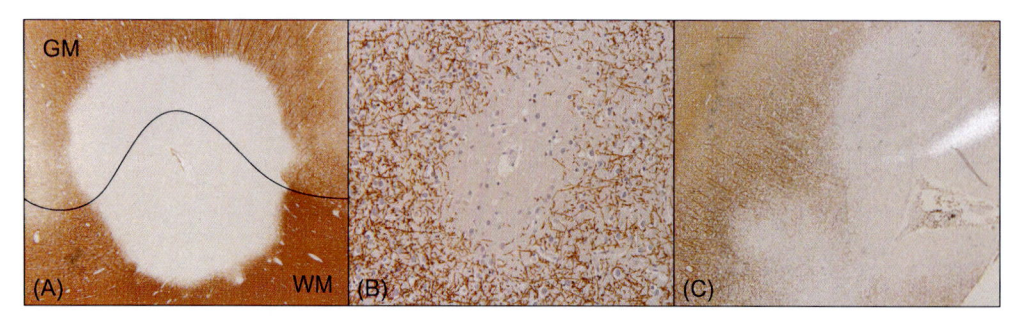

6.7 Cortical grey matter lesions in MS are depicted by their anatomic location. The leucocorticoid lesion (A) is a combined grey and white matter lesion, in which myelin damage affects both the myelin in the white matter (WM) and grey matter (GM). Border of WM and GM shown by line. The intracortical lesion is shown in (B) and subpial lesions (C) show myelin loss in the subpial region. Myelin is stained in all cases for the presence of the myelin proteolipid protein.

pallidum, claustrum amygdala, hypothalamus, substantia nigra, as well as in the spinal cord and frequently involve both the white and grey matter.

Vascular damage and blood–brain barrier

As discussed above, active MS lesions frequently develop around blood vessels, in which alterations in BBB structure and function are observed.[11] In health, the integrity of the BBB is maintained by a network of tight junctions in the endothelial cells together with astrocyte foot processes, while the blood–cerebrospinal fluid barrier is comprised of choroid plexus extensions of the ependymal lining that do not possess BBB properties. In MS, abnormalities in BBB are observed in actively demyelinating lesions as well as in normal-appearing white matter, while no such BBB dysfunction is observed in grey matter lesions.

Acknowledgements

Several of our studies reported in this review have been financially supported by the Netherlands Foundation for MS Research and the Multiple Sclerosis Society of Great Britain and Northern Ireland.

References

1. Compston A. The story of multiple sclerosis. In: Compton A, Ebers G, Lassmann H *et al.* (eds). *McAlpine's Multiple Sclerosis.* London: Churchill Livingstone, 1988: 3–42.
2. Filippi M, Rocca MA, Martino G, *et al.* Magnetization transfer changes in the normal appearing white matter precede the appearance of enhancing lesions in patients with multiple sclerosis. *Ann Neurol* 1998; **43**: 809–14.
3. Allen IV, McKeown SA. A histological, histochemical, and biochemical study of the macroscopically normal white matter in multiple sclerosis. *J Neurol Sci* 1979; **41**: 81–91.
4. Van der Valk P, Amor S. Preactive lesions in multiple sclerosis. *Curr Opin Neurol* 2009; **22**: 207–13.
5. Li H, Newcombe J, Groome N, Cuzner ML. Characterization and distribution of phagocytic macrophages in multiple sclerosis plaques. *Neuropathol Appl Neurobiol* 1993; **19**: 214–23.
6. Dutta R, Trapp BD. Pathogenesis of axonal and neuronal damage in multiple sclerosis. *Neurology* 2007; **68**: S22–31.
7. Raine CS. The Norton Lecture: a review of the oligodendrocyte in the multiple sclerosis lesion. *J Neuroimmunol* 1997; **77**: 135–52.
8. Goldschmidt T, Antel J, König FB, *et al.* Remyelination capacity of the MS brain decreases with disease chronicity. *Neurology* 2009; **72**: 1914–21.
9. Bø L. The histopathology of grey matter demyelination in multiple sclerosis. *Acta Neurol Scand Suppl* 2009; **189**: 51–7.
10. Clarner T, Diederichs F, Berger K, *et al.* Myelin debris regulates inflammatory responses in an experimental demyelination animal model and multiple sclerosis lesions. *Glia* 2012; **60**: 1468–80.
11. Alvarez JI, Cayrol R, Prat A. Disruption of central nervous system barriers in multiple sclerosis. *Biochim Biophys Acta* 2011; **1812**: 252–64.

Part 2 – Animal models

David Baker, Sarah Al-Izki and Katie Lidster

Multiple sclerosis is a uniquely human disease, so animal models can only help us to try and understand disease mechanisms and can sometimes point towards useful therapies. The disease process in MS can probably be split into elements: disease induction, relapsing autoimmunity, demyelination, both immune-dependent and autoimmune-independent neurodegeneration, repair and symptomatic control. These various elements can be modelled in the same or different animals (*Table 6.1*). Current animal models of MS have centred on the induction of demyelination, which was considered to be the pathological hallmark of MS (*Table 6.1*).

Experimental autoimmune encephalomyelitis (EAE) is induced following sensitization to myelin or other nerve proteins. In many mammalian species, including humans, this occurred following vaccinations with preparations containing nerve proteins, for example, the rabies vaccine. Therefore, EAE is clearly not MS but has more features common to MS than any other model system currently described.

Once induced, EAE follows a cascade of events (**6.8**). EAE is an 'outside–in' disease, where disease starts outside the CNS (**6.8**). The 'outside–in' hypothesis has underpinned the concept of myelin-reactive autoimmunity and has shaped the current therapeutic approach to MS. There is also the 'inside–out' hypothesis of MS that starts with oligodendrocyte damage before entry of leucocytes, as may occur in MS. However, oligodendrocyte death alone does not trigger autoimmunity in animals or humans. The brain is not equipped to trigger naive T-cell responses, which probably occur in lymphoid tissues; however, myelin-reactive antibody or viral attack of oligodendrocytes could lead to induction of stress proteins such as α-B crystallin to which humans respond.

Autoimmunity is a product of circumstance and a polygenic response. Likewise, autoimmunity in animals is polygenic and requires lymphocytes to break free from the homeostatic control mechanisms that maintain immune tolerance to self and thereby prevent autoimmunity from developing. In animals, this is achieved using strong adjuvants to boost the number of autoreactive lymphocytes. Once this has occurred any signal that stimulates cells to change their phenotype, such that they can then circulate into tissues, can trigger disease. This occurs once they enter the CNS and find their specific antigenic target (**6.8**).

Lymphocyte binding to and extravasation into the CNS is an early feature of lesion formation (**6.9**). These cells then trigger paralytic disease, which is associated with BBB dysfunction (**6.10**) and mononuclear cell perivascular infiltration of the CNS, as seen in MS (**6.11**). This induces a reversible conduction block resulting in ascending paralysis from the tail to hindlimbs and occasionally the forelimbs. The cells may subsequently invade the parenchyma and result in demyelination and neuroaxonal loss (**6.12**). Remyelination often ensues but chronically demyelinated and gliotic lesions can be induced. Demyelination and progressive neuronal

Table 6.1 Models of demyelination	
Route to demyelination approach	**Chief role of model**
Myelin mutants	Myelin formation*
Oligodendrocyte toxins	Study oligodendrocyte
	Function and promotion of myelin repair*
Glia trophic viral attack	Viral trigger of autoimmunity (cross-reactive immunity)
Experimental autoimmune encephalomyelitis	Autoimmunity, neuroprotection, repair, symptom control*

*These models have shown that neurodegeneration can occur following established dysmyelination or demyelination and so may also have the potential to model elements of progressive MS that does not respond to immunosuppression.

Pathology of multiple sclerosis part 2 – animal models

loss develops in some strains and species, depending on the immunizing antigen.

The neurological course varies depending on the inducing antigen and the species and strain of animal used. The C57BL/6 mouse, often used in transgenic animal experiments, usually develops a monophasic attack due to the severity of the immune attack and degree of nerve loss, and shows chronic or non-remitting paresis. Other strains such as SJL and ABH mice can be induced to develop a relapsing and secondary progressive phenotype that

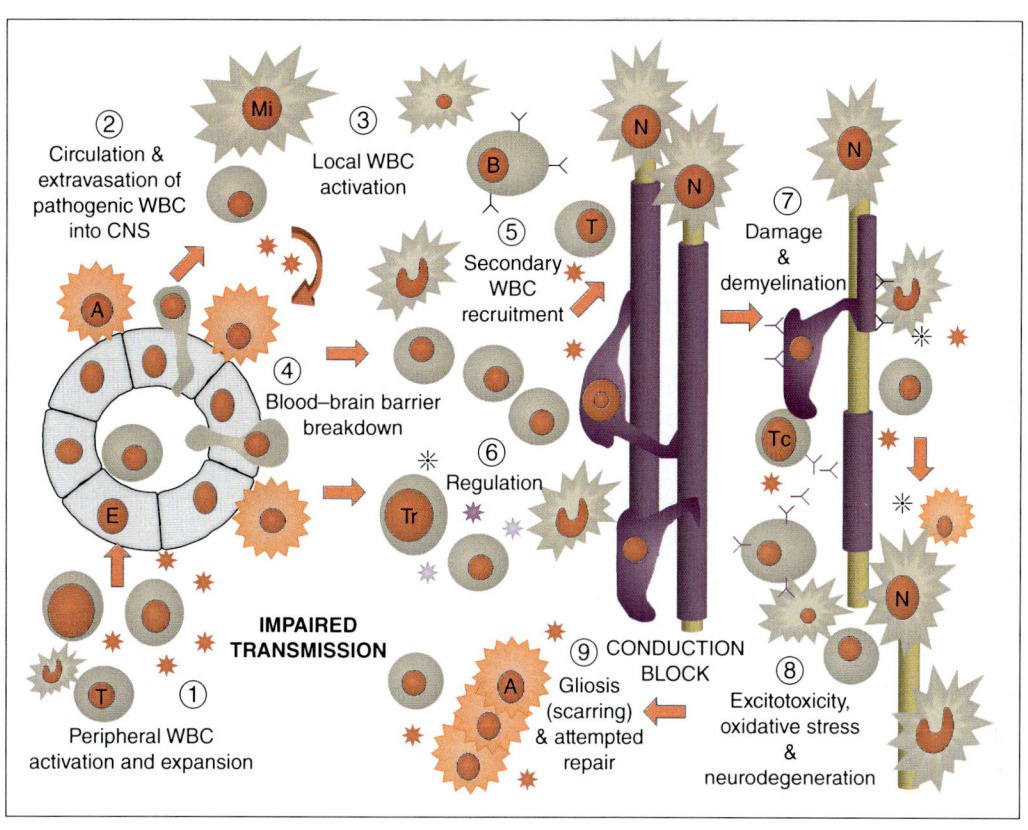

6.8 Cascade of pathological events in experimental autoimmune encephalomyelitis. WBC, white blood cell.

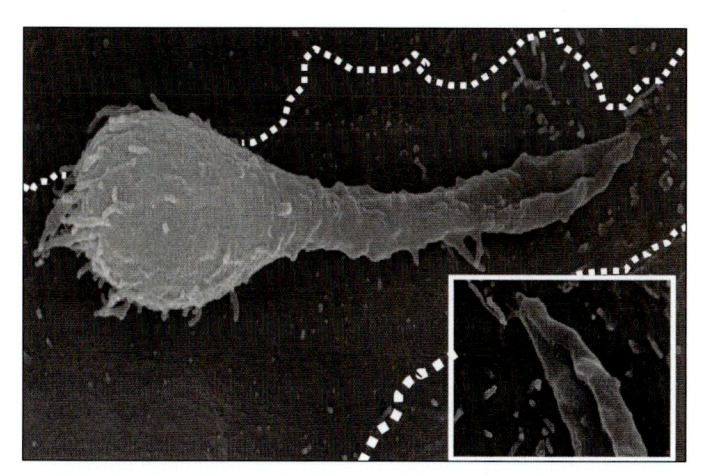

6.9 Scanning electron micrograph showing a leucocyte migrating through the blood vessel near the endothelial cell (*dotted line*) junction during experimental autoimmune encephalomyelitis.

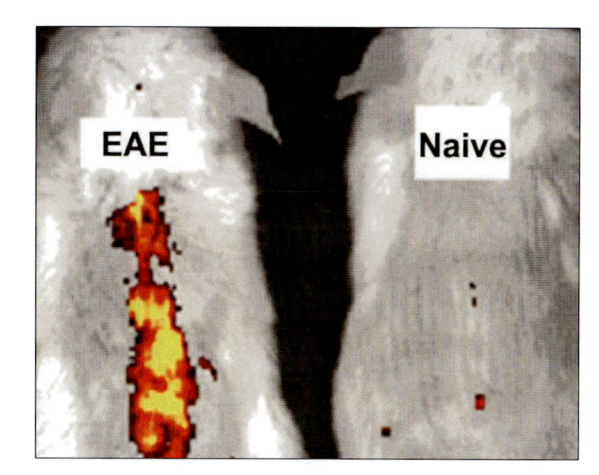

6.10 Blood–brain barrier dysfunction during active experimental autoimmune encephalomyelitis. Bioluminesence of a fluorescent albumin probe injected into a healthy mouse and a mouse with experimental autoimmune encephalomyelitis. There is active accumulation in the spinal cord but not the brain in a mouse with hindlimb and tail paralysis during active relapse.

develops over several months. Likewise, the Lewis rat usually develops a single attack with good recovery, whereas the DA rat relapses. Disease in EAE is usually concentrated in the spinal cord (**6.10**). Although there is often grey matter involvement, myelin-induced EAE disease is concentrated in the white matter (**6.12**). These lesions can occur anywhere in the CNS; for example, in the optic nerve the lesion results in retinal ganglion cell loss and visual dysfunction (**6.13**). Brain lesions can and do occur and commonly develop in the marmoset, which is a non-human primate. In all instances the disease is driven by the action of T cells and can occur in the absence of mature B-cell responses (**6.8**). However, B-cell and autoantibody responses contribute to pathology by stimulating T cells and through targeted destruction of myelin and nerves; an antibody response to myelin or nerve proteins typically leads to complement activation and the opsonization of nerve structures for attack by macrophages/microglia and interference with nerve or axonal function.

It is relatively easy to decipher the content of studies in EAE and this can be seen by looking at the neurological course (**6.14**) before reading the — often inflated — claims in many studies. If the treatment arm shows a delay and/or reduction in the severity of disease at its peak, then this is generally identifying an immunosuppressive effect (**6.13**). It will therefore follow that there will be less immune infiltration of the CNS, notably in the spinal cord, and there will be less downstream consequences of this. This will mean that there will be fewer inflammatory cells and hence fewer proinflammatory cytokines, less demyelination and less nerve cell and axonal loss. If there is only modest influence on disease course as a minor delay or attenuation of disease as found in many EAE studies, it would be questionable whether this would equate to a meaningful outcome in MS, but is often sufficient to allow the publication of the work. However, even if a therapy provides very effective immunosuppression that inhibits all relapsing disease this is only indirect neuroprotection, because the damaging autoimmune response never arrived in the CNS in the first place. However, if a compound is neuroprotective but not immunosuppressive, you will not see any influence on the initiation of disease but you will see more effective recovery, which equates to less nerve loss (**6.14**).

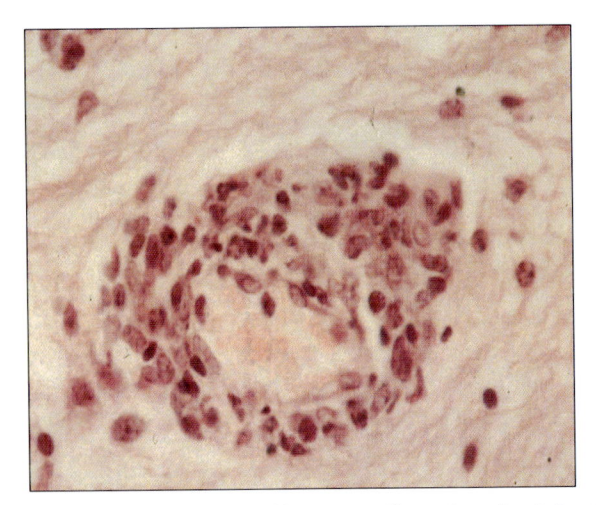

6.11 Perivascular cell lesion. Haematoxylin and eosin stain of spinal cord.

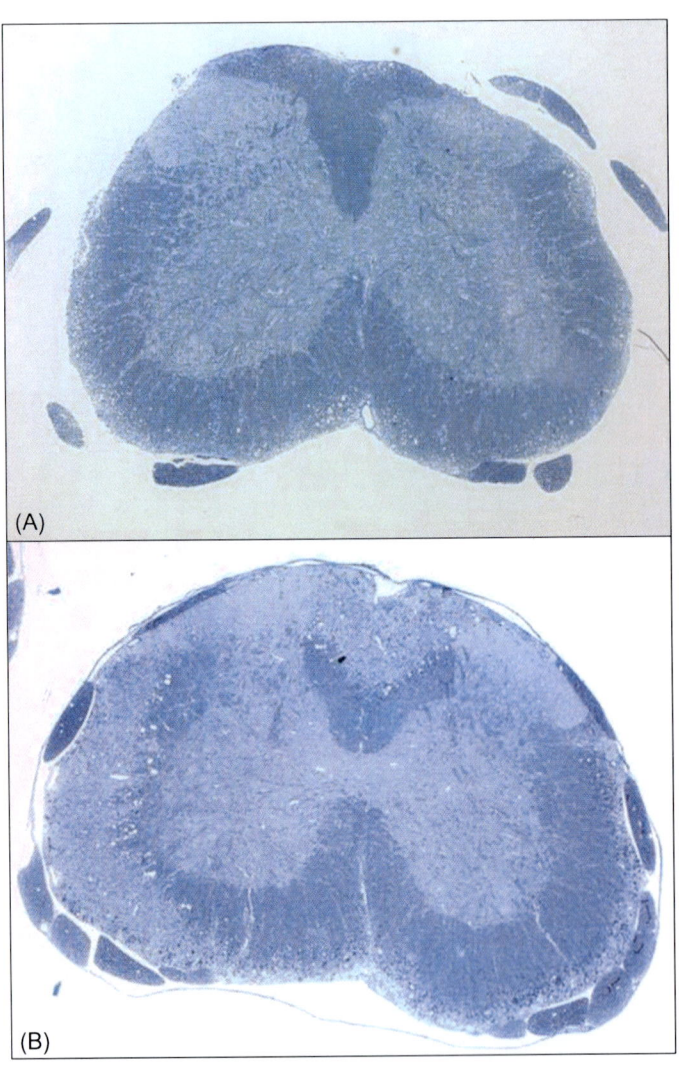

6.12 Loss of myelin in an autoimmune model of MS. Spinal cord after (A) one attack with limited nerve damage or (B) four attacks with extensive myelin loss (*dark blue*) and nerves. The dorsal and lateral column is severely affected. The peripheral nerve roots (*dark blue on the outer edge of the spinal cord*) show no involvement (*Toluidine blue stain*).

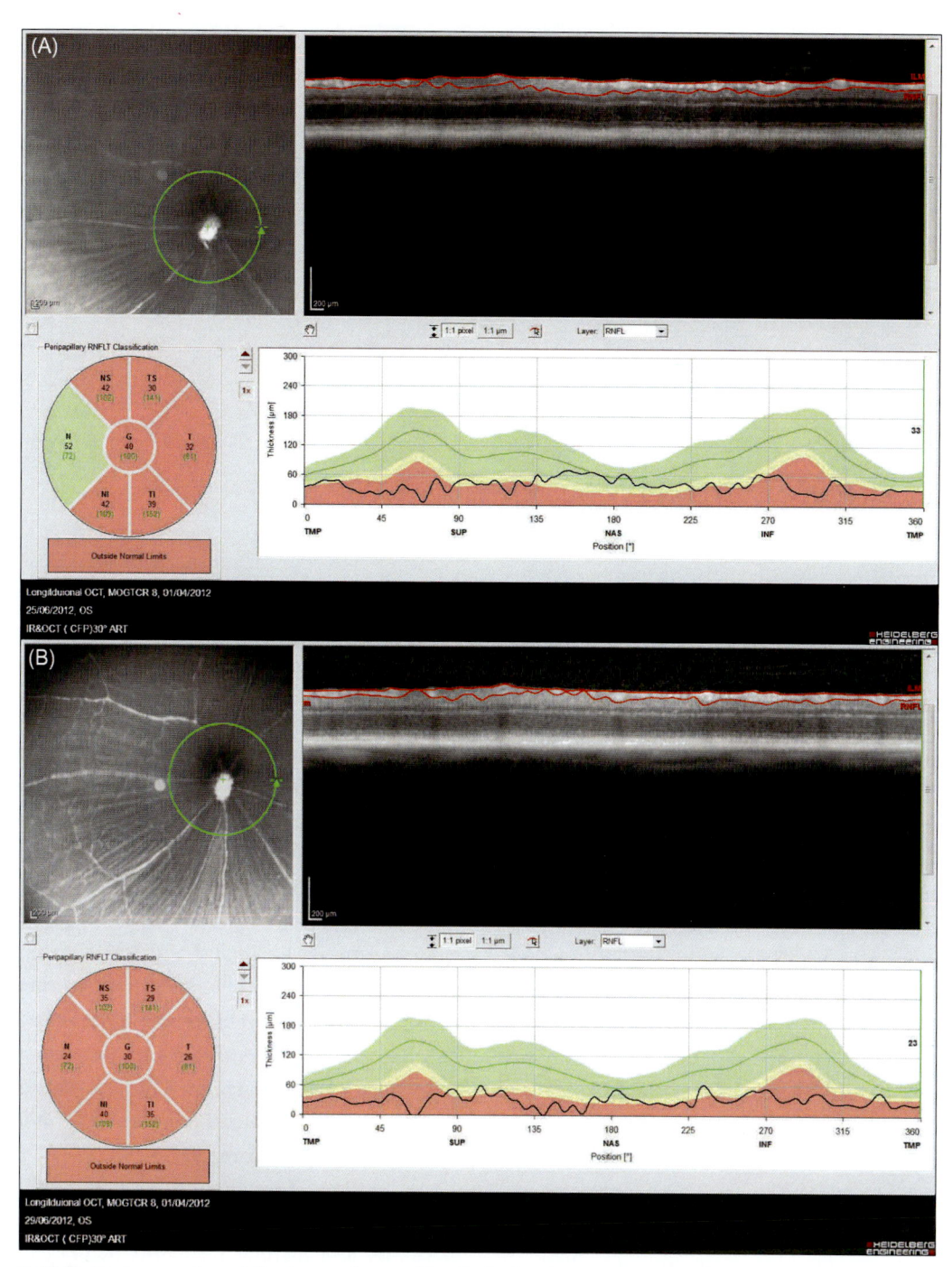

6.13 Retinal nerve loss following optic neuritis. Optical coherence tomography scan of the retinal nerve fibre layer (RNFL) in myelin-specific T-cell receptor transgenic C57BL/6 mouse before (A) and after (B) the development of optic neuritis. The RNFL thickness (*highlighted in red*) was assessed in the retina surrounding the optic nerve head (*green circles*). The nasal quadrant RNFL thickness was reduced from 52 μM to 24 μM, while the temporal quadrant reduced from 32 μM to 26 μM.

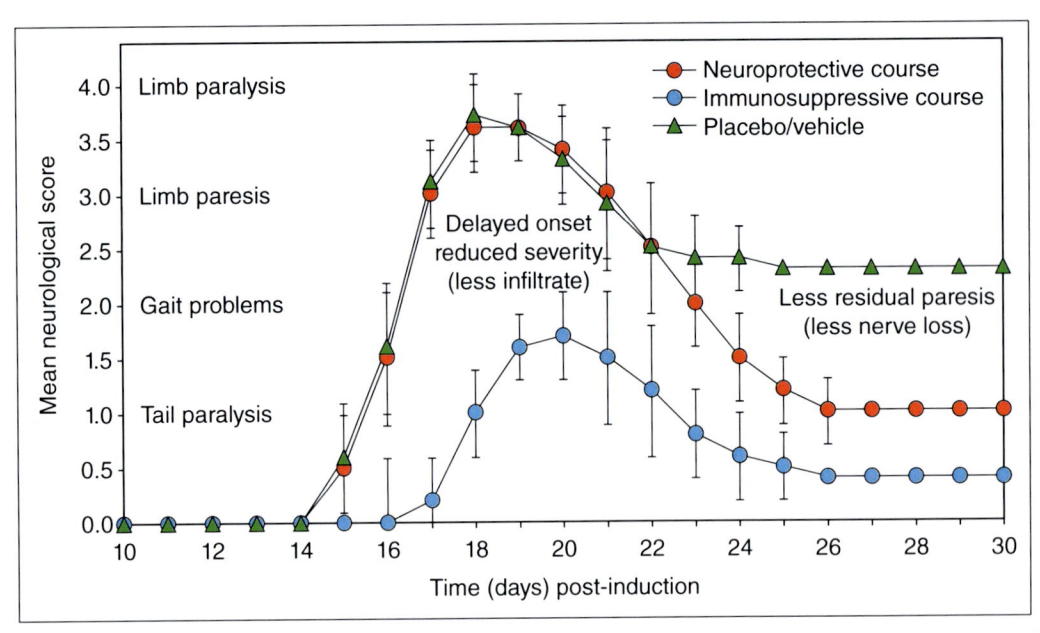

6.14 Understanding the data of rodent neurological scores in experimental autoimmune encephalomyelitis.

There has been a poor rate of translation of treatments from animal models into treatments for people with MS. This may have something to do with the models themselves but importantly it has a lot to do with how they are used and how the information from them is applied. It should also be said that poor or suboptimal trial design in MS has contributed to this failure. The vast majority of studies in EAE concern themselves with understanding autoimmune mechanisms rather than attempting to find effective therapies. As such, most studies apply treatments before disease is induced, as a prophylactic treatment, which clearly would not be feasible in MS. Very few animal studies initiate treatments after the first attack. Furthermore, despite the differences in drug metabolism between animals and humans, few studies in MS use doses anywhere near those used in animals that were used to justify the trials. However, if common disease mechanisms are targeted there is a good chance of success. More and more treatments that were initially shown to be effective in relapsing EAE are translating into drugs to control relapsing MS, a phase of the disease that is immune-mediated (**6.8**).

However, even in these simple autoimmune models it is clear that once sufficient damage has accumulated, autoimmune-independent neurodegenerative processes are initiated that no longer respond to immunosuppression (**6.15**). This non-relapsing progression is probably mediated by factors produced by the glial response (**6.16**) that target vulnerable demyelinated nerves (**6.15**). Therefore, a disease that is indeed autoimmune in nature can result in progressive disability that does not respond to immunosuppression, which occurs in progressive MS. This would argue for early and aggressive treatment of MS and suggests that neuroprotective as well as immunomodulatory approaches are required for the more effective treatment of MS. The ability to control the immune response allows one to explore repair strategies. The use of chemically induced re/demyelination animal models has helped identify a number of targets for repair.

As animals lose neural circuitry (**6.12**), progressive disability develops and additional signs such as a tremor, spasticity and bladder problems (**6.17**) can develop. These can be used as a tool to examine symptomatic control agents.

It can therefore be seen that animal models can provide an insight into MS pathogenesis and treatment efficacy, due to features that these models have in common with human disease.

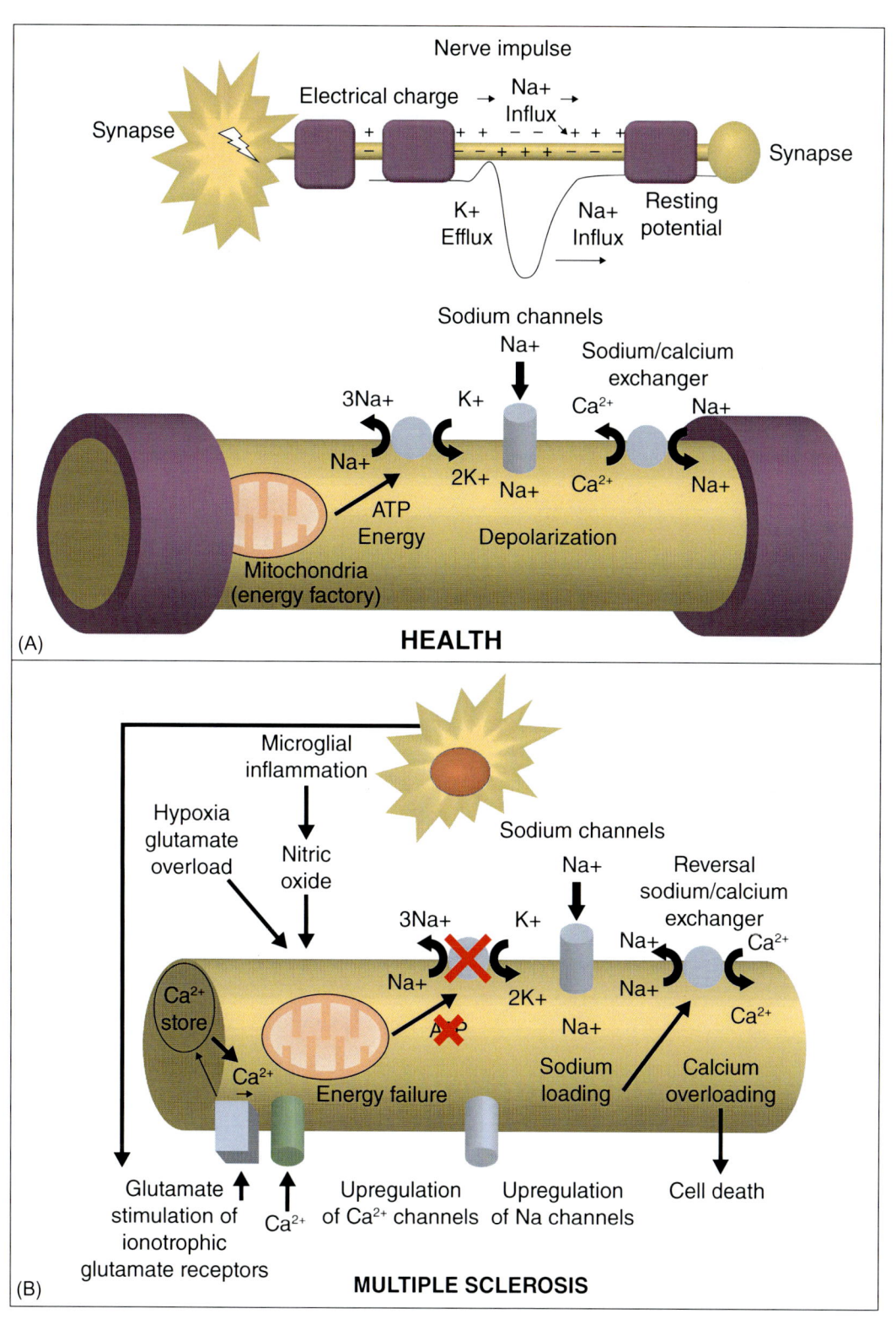

6.15 Adaptive immune response-independent neurodegeneration for progressive neurological deficit. (A) This is a putative mechanism that may contribute to progressive MS. (B) Following demyelination, ion channels redistribute to maintain nerve function. In the presence of a glial response, mitochondrial energy deficits lead to the block of ion pumps that lead to sodium and calcium loading following reversal of the ion exchanger, which can trigger cell death.

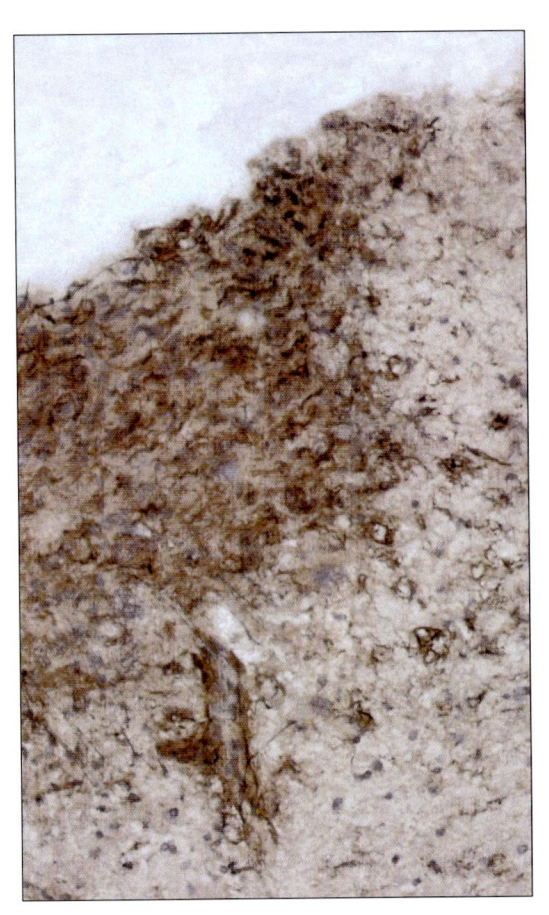

6.16 Activated microglia in a chronic experimental autoimmune encephalomyelitis lesion. Microglia on the edge of chronic long-established EAE lesions were stained by macrophage-specific antibodies using immunoperoxidase.

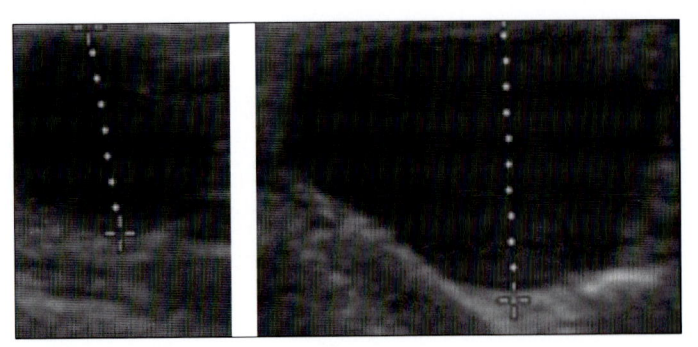

6.17 Ultrasound showing bladder distension during EAE.

Further reading

1. Al-Izki S, Pryce G, O'Neill JK, Butter C, Giovannoni G, Baker D. Practical guide to the induction of relapsing progressive experimental autoimmune encephalomyelitis in the Biozzi ABH mouse. *Mult Scler Relat Disord* 2012; **1**: 29–38.
2. Baker D, Gerritsen W, Rundle J, Amor S. Critical appraisal of animal models of multiple sclerosis. *Mult Scler J* 2011; **17**: 647–57.
3. Baker D, Amor S. Publication guidelines for refereeing and reporting on animal use in experimental autoimmune encephalomyelitis. *J Neuroimmunol* 2012; **242**: 78–83.

Chapter 7

Treatment issues in multiple sclerosis

Monica Marta and Maria Papachatzaki

Introduction

There are three types of treatment that are used in MS:

1. **Symptomatic therapies.** These address acute or residual symptoms caused by MS; examples include: baclofen or tizanidine for spasticity; modafinil or amantadine for fatigue; and gabapentin, pregabalin or carbamazepine for pain. The use of symptomatic therapies is discussed in more detail in Chapter 9.
2. **Treatment for relapses.** The mainstay of relapse treatment is high-dose methylprednisolone (usually 0.5–1 g intravenous methylprednisolone for 3–5 days but 500 mg oral methylprednisolone per day for 5 days is an alternative); this reduces the relapse duration by causing apoptosis of inflammatory cells and stabilization of the BBB. Administration of high-dose methylprednisolone should occur within 2 weeks of the relapse symptom onset to ensure optimal efficacy. It is important to ensure that concurrent infection (such as urinary tract infection) and other factors potentially worsened by steroid administration, such as gastritis or recurrent herpes infections, are treated prophylactically. The evidence that steroids alter long-term outcomes in MS is weak and inconsistent.
3. **Disease-modifying drugs (DMDs).** These are taken on a regular basis (daily, every other day, three times per week, weekly, monthly or yearly) to reduce the number of relapses and improve long-term disability-related outcomes in MS. The ultimate objective for these drugs is to abolish clinical and MRI evidence of disease activity; as yet the evidence supporting either neuroprotective or neuroregenerative effects from licensed therapies is speculative.

The **first-line DMDs** have been available for over 15 years and have an extremely good safety profile but moderate average efficacy. They are all administered by injection, albeit self-administered; different formulations have different attributes. Furthermore, the relatively common and unpleasant post-injection reactions deter a number of people from either choosing or adhering to the treatment.

Second-line DMDs have significantly better efficacy, both in terms of a significant reduction in relapse rate and delay in disease progression. However, national guidelines, for example those produced by the National Institute for Health and Clinical Excellence (NICE) in the UK, have restricted their use. In the UK, natalizumab is restricted to those patients with 'highly active disease', and fingolimod to those patients who have failed (i.e. relapsed while taking) interferon (IFN)-β. These drugs have a significant risk profile, with an increased risk of opportunistic infections and possibly tumours, which likely occur as a result of immunosuppression. A general rule is that the more effective the drug is, the more serious the potential side effects.

There are two contrasting strategies that can be used when deciding which therapy to use in a patient with active MS. The most commonly used strategy is to start with a first-line DMD and to monitor response to treatment. If the first-line therapy fails to suppress inflammatory activity, then the patient can be switched to a second-line treatment. This is the strategy that the UK regulatory authorities have supported; safety concerns are paramount.

The second strategy, which has primarily been used in clinical trials to date, is to initiate treatment early with a drug(s) with high immunosuppressive effects in an attempt to reset or reboot the immune system. This has shown promising results, although, so far, the number of patients treated is relatively low and follow-up is relatively short. This approach is commonly referred to as 'induction therapy'.

To date there are no available treatments that have been shown to alter the course of progressive MS without relapses.

First-line disease-modifying drugs

IFN-β and glatiramer acetate (GA) reduce relapse rates and MRI evidence of disease activity (new T2 lesions and gadolinium-enhancing (Gd+) lesions) in MS. MRI activity is considered a surrogate marker of disease activity, even if the relationship between MRI lesion load, relapse frequency and disability in MS and clinically isolated syndrome is not clearly defined. It must be noted that the outcome measures currently used for evaluating treatment efficacy are unsatisfactory.

In people with either RRMS or SPMS with relapses, both IFN-β and GA reduce relapse rates by approximately a third over 2 years. People with clinically isolated syndrome who have an abnormal MRI, indicating a high probability of conversion to MS, and those who subsequently meet the revised McDonald criteria for MS also qualify for treatment with IFN-β and/or GA. In people with clinically isolated syndrome, the conversion rate to clinically definitive MS falls from 45–50% to 28–35% over 2–3 years in those taking IFN-β or GA compared to those who do not receive treatment.

IFN-β and GA may reduce the development of disability through relapse prevention; however, there is currently no evidence that they reduce disability progression unrelated to relapses.

Interferon-β

IFN-β reduces the activation and proliferation of inflammatory cells and production of inflammatory cytokines in peripheral blood and CSF; it also stabilizes the BBB. As mentioned above, the use of IFN-β is limited to some degree by its side effects. The most commonly encountered side effects include the following.

1. Flu-like symptoms occurring within hours of each dose and lasting for up to 3 days. These symptoms often improve within weeks to months. They can be ameliorated by the prophylactic use of paracetamol and/or ibuprofen and injecting at night-time; in some patients the mild pyrexia that occurs because of IFN-β injections can cause temporary conduction block (see Chapter 5) and worsen pre-existing neurological deficits.
2. Injection-site reactions. These are inflamed areas that usually disappear within a few weeks. They can be prevented to some degree by rotating the site of injection; making sure injection fluid is at room temperature before injection and cooling the site of injection before and/or after injection; and using an aseptic technique. Injection-site reactions are generally less common with intramuscular injections than with subcutaneous ones; the commonest injection-site reaction seen with intramuscular injections is a small bruise. Very occasionally, there may be aseptic skin necrosis, which may require surgical treatment.
3. Lymphopenia and liver dysfunction. On rare occasions, the latter has been documented to progress to hepatic failure. Monitoring for both of these is initially performed regularly, but if blood tests are persistently normal then the frequency of monitoring can be reduced. If abnormal liver function tests (LFT) and/or moderate/severe lymphopenia are found, the dose of IFN-β should be titrated down.
4. Patients with pre-existing monoclonal gammopathies are at risk for systemic capillary leak syndrome, and therefore all patients should be screened for monoclonal gammopathy before starting IFN-β.
5. Depression and suicidal ideation can occur in people with MS and may be worsened by IFN-β; however, there is no evidence that IFN-β causes these symptoms.
6. Neutralizing antibodies (NAbs) to IFN-β develop in approximately 20% of patients; the rate varies depending on the formulation used. NAbs typically develop towards the end of the first year of treatment with a peak incidence at approximately 2 years. NAbs abrogate the effects of IFN-β and are an indication for either stopping or switching treatment.

There are accepted safety measures that should be followed when initiating a patient on IFN-β. A full blood count (FBC), LFT and serum immunoelectrophoresis should be performed before starting treatment, and FBC and LFT repeated at 1 month, 3 months and 6 months after starting treatment, and then every 6 months after this. Women are advised against becoming pregnant and breast-feeding while on IFN-β.

Clinical or brain MRI activity during the first year of IFN-β is an indicator of a poor response to treatment and may prompt a change in treatment.

There are a number of different formulations of IFN-β, all of which are used in clinical practice. However, these have subtle differences, in terms of both the active compound and route and frequency of administration.

Interferon-β1b: Betaferon® and Extavia® (7.1, 7.2, 7.3)

The active compound (and excipient) is the same in both drugs. It is made in *Escherichia coli* cell lines; the cytokine has

Treatment issues in multiple sclerosis 53

a single nucleotide modification from naturally occurring human IFN-β (serine substituted for cysteine at residue 17) and this is then purified to a powder. The 250 μg (8.0 million IU) in 1 ml is administered as a subcutaneous injection every other day. The powder formulation needs to be reconstituted (mixed with saline) before injection, thus avoiding the need for refrigerator storage.

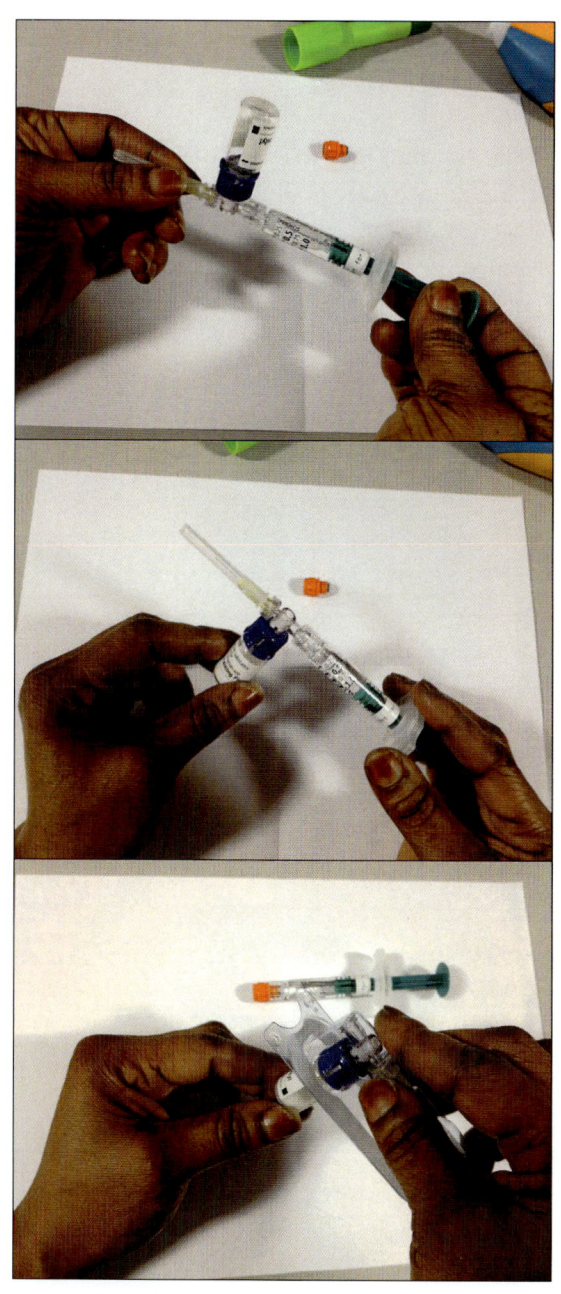

7.1 Betaferon® preparation of solution.

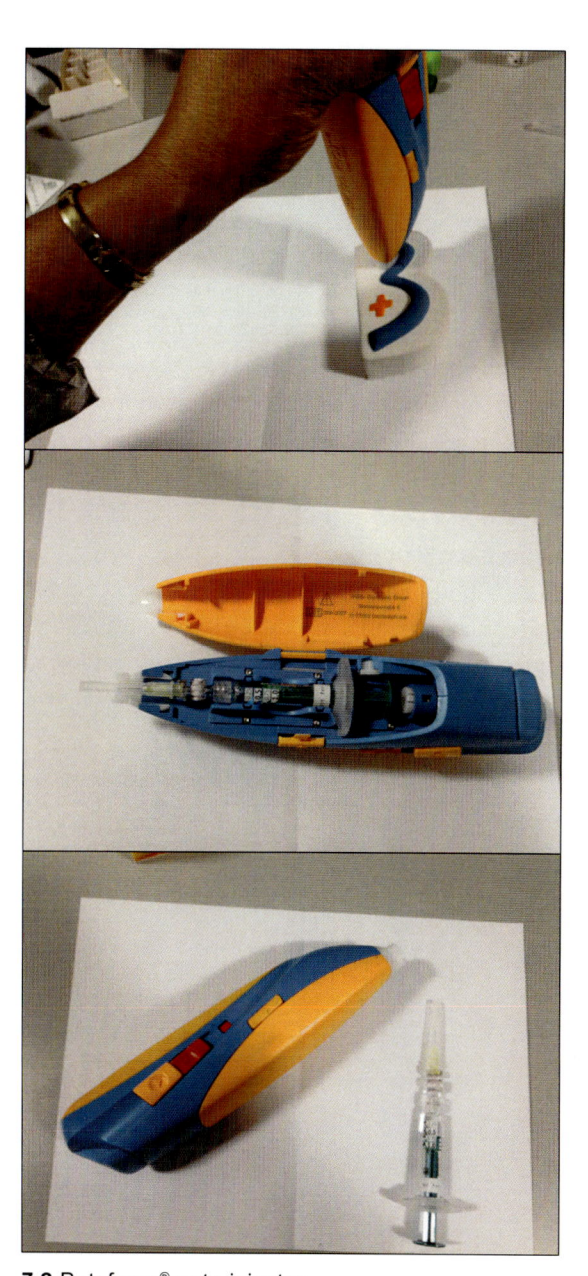

7.2 Betaferon® auto-injector.

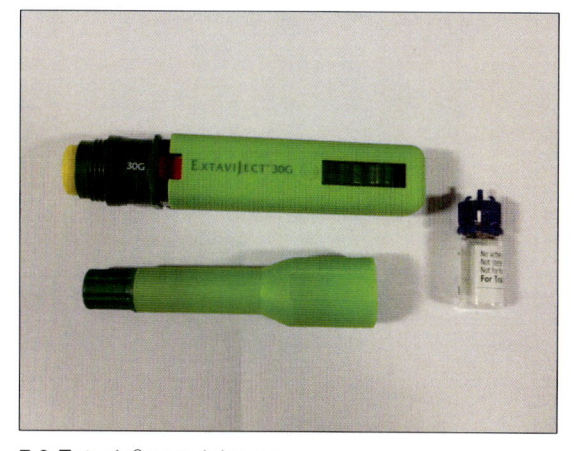

7.3 Extavia® auto-injector.

Interferon-β1a: Avonex® and Rebif®

This protein is the naturally occurring IFN-β. It is produced in CHO (Chinese hamster ovary) cell lines, where it acquires the mammalian post-translation modifications, unlike the IFN-β synthesized in *E. coli*.

Avonex® is dispensed in premixed syringes with 30 μg (6 MIU) of IFN-β1a in 0.5 ml of solution, and is administered once weekly as an intramuscular injection (**7.4**, **7.5**). It should be stored refrigerated at 2–5°C, but is stable at room temperature for up to 1 week. A solution for injections and a powder formulation are also available, with the latter being useful for travel, as refrigeration is not required.

Rebif® is injected at a dose of 44 μg (12 MIU) of IFN-β1a in 1.0 ml solution three times per week subcutaneously (**7.6**, **7.7**). The devices (RebiSmart or RebiSlide), which contain a prefilled cartridge must be stored in a refrigerator, but they are stable for a single period of up to 14 days at room temperature.

Glatiramer acetate: Copaxone®

Copaxone® is the acetate salt of synthetic polypeptides, containing four naturally occurring amino acids found in myelin: L-glutamic acid, L-alanine, L-tyrosine and L-lysine, in determined molar fraction ranges. Copaxone® is produced as 20-mg GA in 1 ml of solution and is given subcutaneously once daily (**7.8**).

The mechanism of action is unknown. The proposed mechanisms include partial activation and tolerance induction of myelin basic protein-specific T cells and induction of GA-reactive T-helper-2-like regulatory T cells; the other mechanisms that have been described do not appear to be relevant *in vivo*.

The side effects are different to those seen with IFN-β. Side effects that patients should be warned about when starting therapy include the following.

1. Vasodilatation (flushing), chest tightness, dyspnoea, palpitations and/or tachycardia, which occur immediately following injection. These symptoms tend to be short-lived and resolve spontaneously. They are unpredictable and occur infrequently.

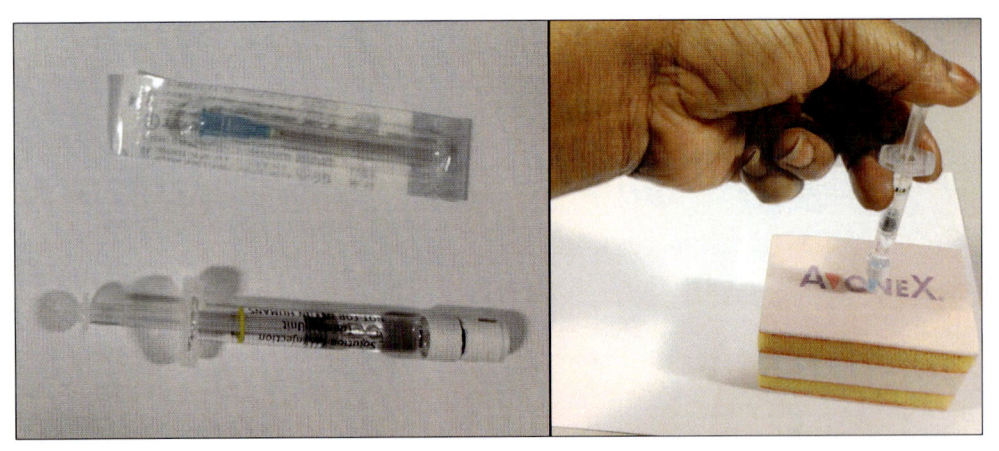

7.4 Avonex® pre-mixed syringes.

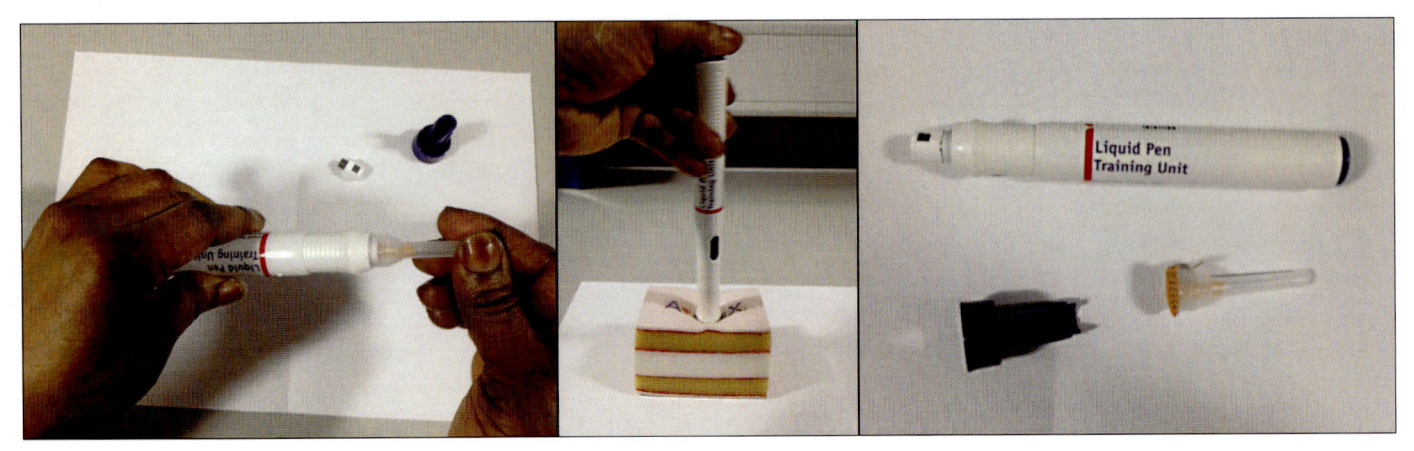

7.5 Avonex® auto-injector.

2. Convulsions and/or anaphylactoid or allergic reactions have all been reported; however, these are extremely rare.
3. In those patients with pre-existing renal impairment, there is a suggestion that Copaxone may worsen renal function. Therefore, in those with pre-existing renal disease renal function should be monitored on treatment.
4. Lipoatrophy may be seen at injection sites. This is seen more frequently than with IFN-β. It is often persistent and commonly precipitates a change of treatment.
5. Pseudolymphoma. Enlarged, painful and tender regional lymph nodes draining the site of injection. Lymph node biopsy reveals non-specific reactive nodes.

If the prefilled syringes cannot be kept in a refrigerator, they can be stored once at room temperature for up to 1 month.

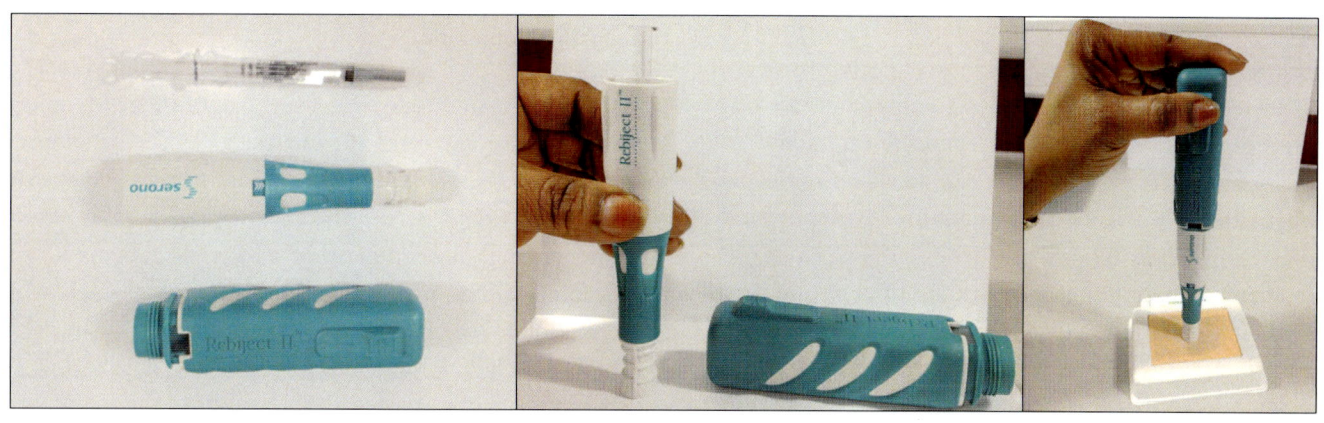

7.6 Rebif® auto-injector: Rebiject II.

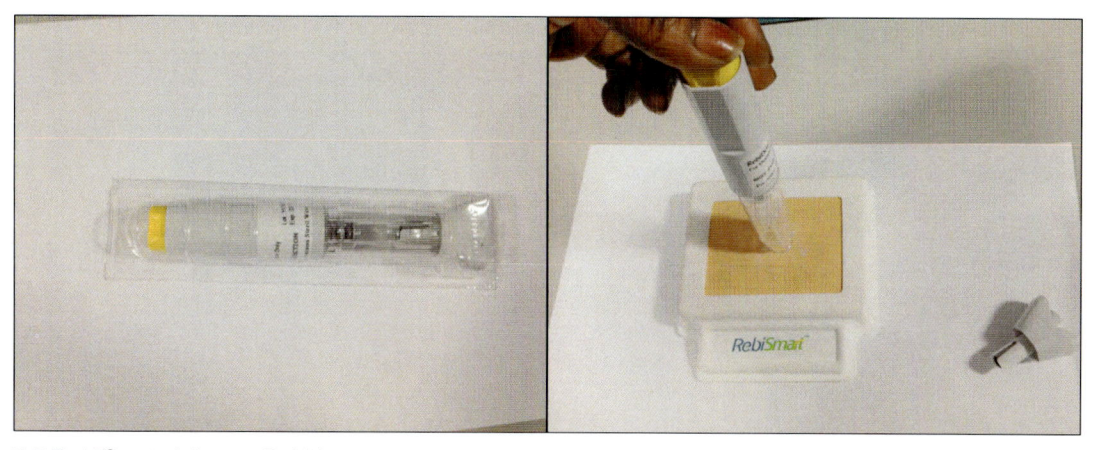

7.7 Rebif® auto-injector: Rebidose pen.

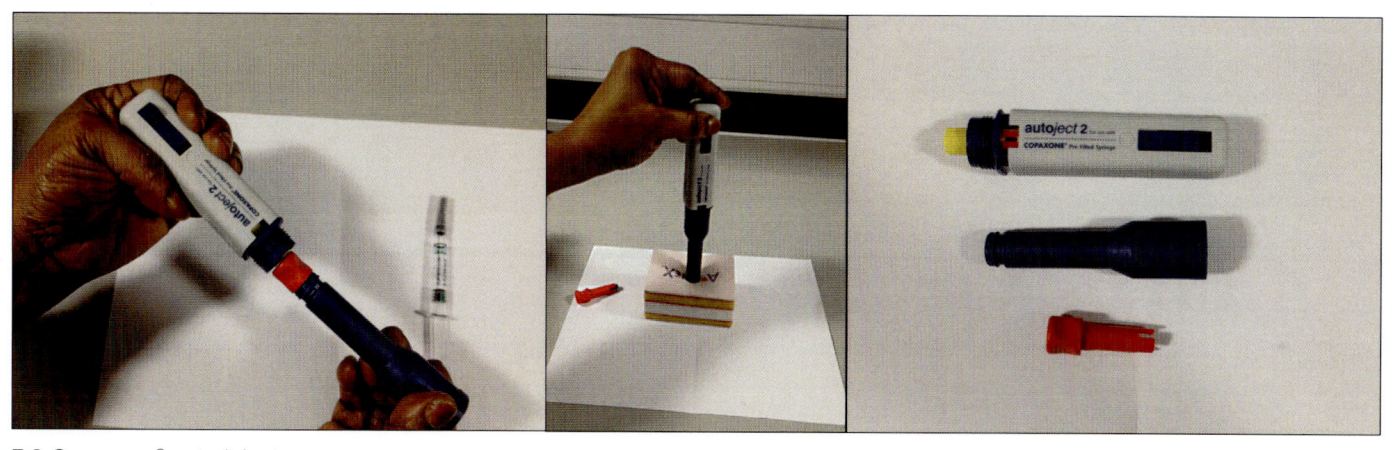

7.8 Copaxone® auto-injector.

Second-line disease-modifying therapy

For situations where first-line treatments have failed or have stopped providing any benefit, a variety of second-line treatments exist. These have either been approved in the past few years, or are currently under evaluation by the regulatory authorities.

Natalizumab (Tysabri®)

Natalizumab is a monoclonal antibody that inhibits lymphocyte and monocyte migration across the BBB, thereby reducing effector inflammatory mechanisms in the CNS. It selectively binds to the α4 subunit of the α4β1-integrin on leucocytes, blocking leucocyte interaction with the endothelial receptor vascular cell adhesion molecule 1. Through this, it prevents the initiation of lymphocyte and monocyte migration across the BBB into the CNS.

Natalizumab is approved as a monotherapy in patients with RRMS with highly active disease in both treatment-naïve patients and those who have demonstrated a poor response to first-line treatment. It is administered intravenously once monthly at a dose of 300 mg.

Natalizumab has been shown to reduce the annualized relapse rate by 68–70%; reduce the number of new or enlarging T2 lesions by 82%; reduce the number of Gd+ lesions by over 92%; and reduce the risk of sustained Expanded Disability Status Score (EDSS) progression by 42% compared to placebo. At present a phase III study is being performed in patients with SPMS (ASCEND).[1]

Natalizumab has a number of relatively common side effects in addition to rare but serious side effects related to the compartment-specific immunosuppression caused by its mechanism of action.

1. Infusion-related reactions such as headache, allergic hypersensitivity (rash or urticaria) occur in approximately 4% of patients and more serious anaphylactoid reactions occur in approximately 1%, usually due to the development of NAbs (see below) (**7.9**). Serological abnormalities such as abnormal LFT, which are monitored for periodically, occur rarely. Increased blood levels of lymphocytes, monocytes, eosinophils and basophils occur as a result of the shift of the marginating pool of white blood cells into the central compartment.

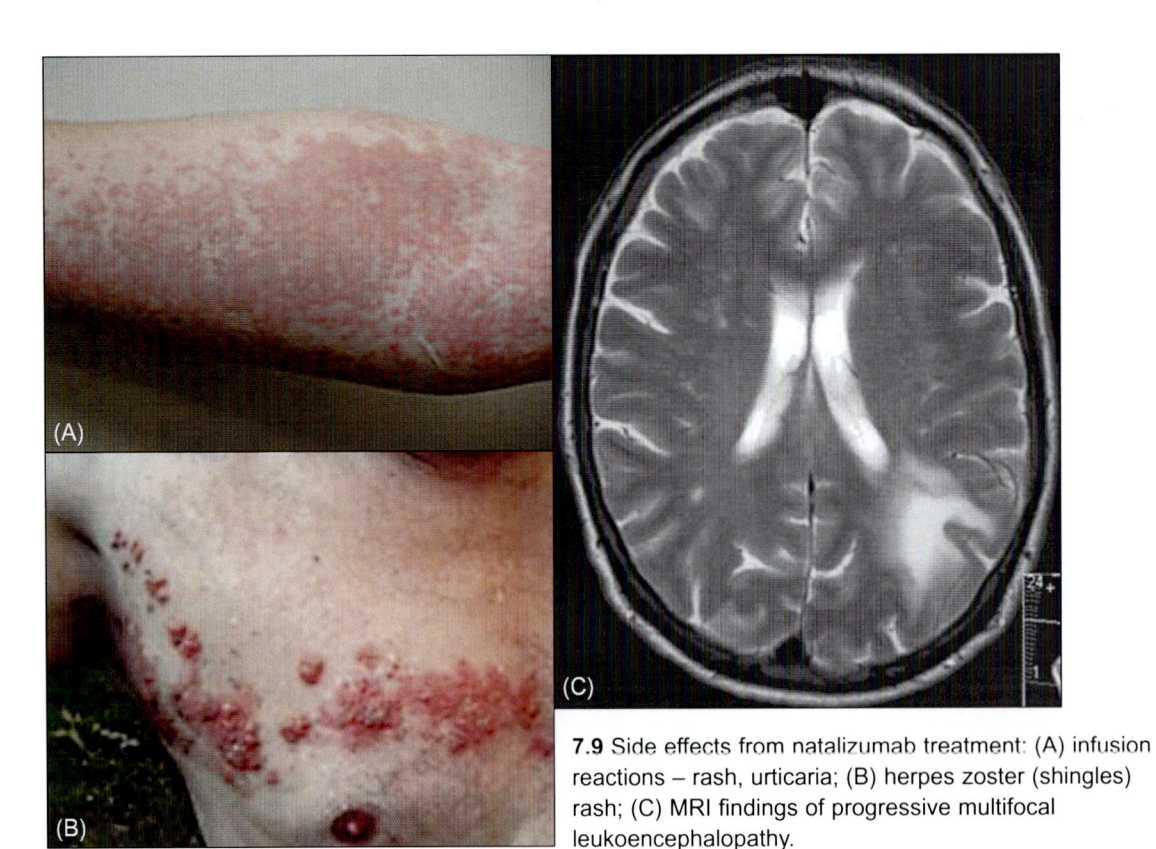

7.9 Side effects from natalizumab treatment: (A) infusion reactions – rash, urticaria; (B) herpes zoster (shingles) rash; (C) MRI findings of progressive multifocal leukoencephalopathy.

Treatment issues in multiple sclerosis

2. Infections, including respiratory, urinary tract and herpes infections, have been seen at a slightly higher rate in those patients treated with natalizumab in clinical trials.
3. NAbs: 8–10% of patients with MS treated with natalizumab develop NAbs that can interfere with clinical and MRI efficacy. NAbs can be either transient or persistent, and are strongly linked to the occurrence of infusion reactions: 75% of those patients who have infusion reactions are antibody positive. Patients who are persistently Nab positive should be advised to discontinue treatment. NAbs should be measured routinely after 12 months of treatment.

The main serious adverse event associated with natalizumab therapy is progressive multifocal leukoencephalopathy (PML). PML is a severe demyelinating disease of the CNS, which is caused by reactivation of the JC virus (JCV; a human polyomavirus) within the CNS compartment. This virus causes a persistent infection in about 60% of the general adult population. The reactivation of JCV has been associated with the use of immunosuppressive therapies. The risk of PML varies over time, and is related to three main factors (**7.10**).

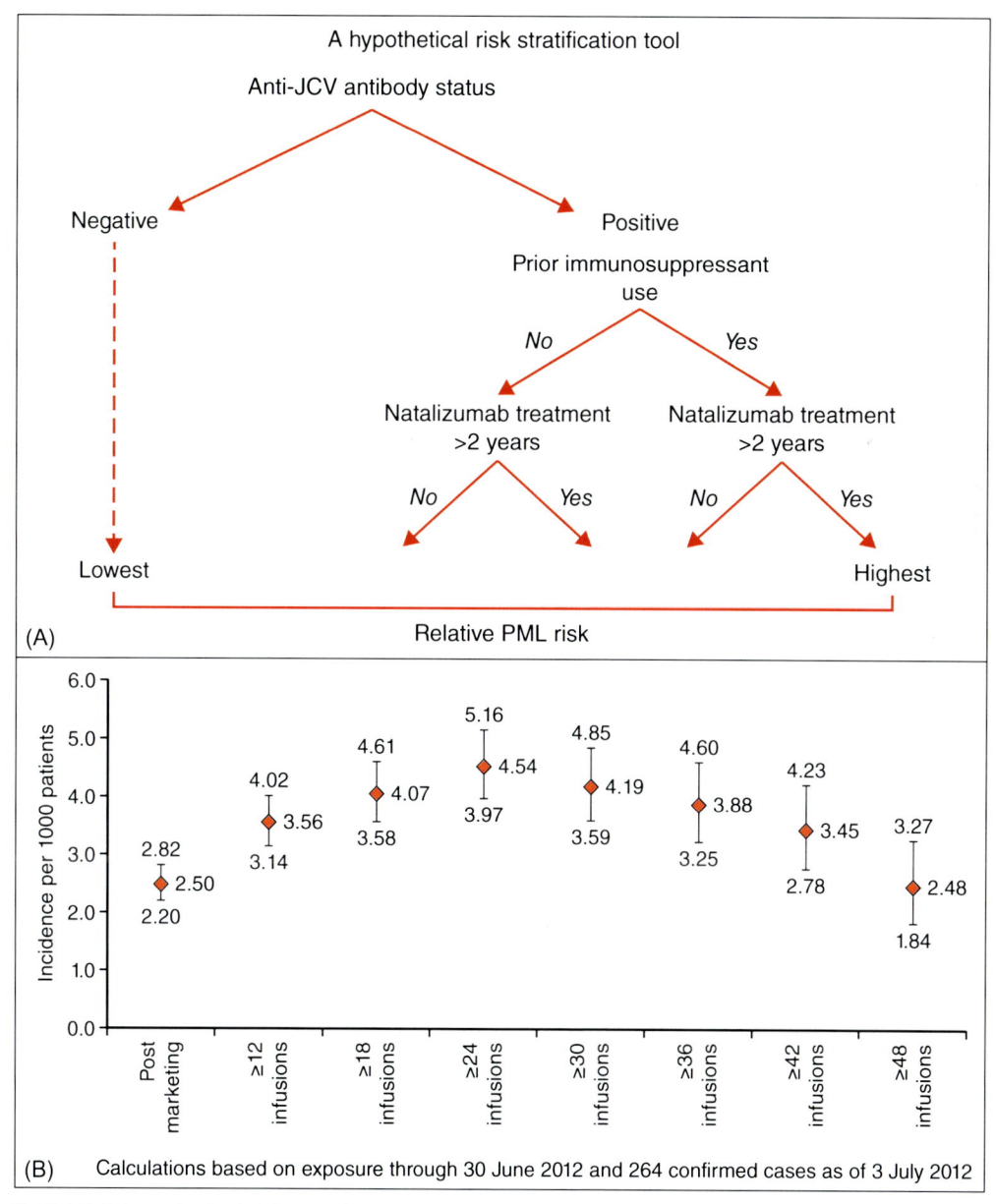

7.10 (A) A hypothetical risk stratification tool to enable discussion of progressive multifocal leukoencephalopathy (PML) risk. (B) PML risk estimates by natalizumab treatment duration.

58 Treatment issues in multiple sclerosis

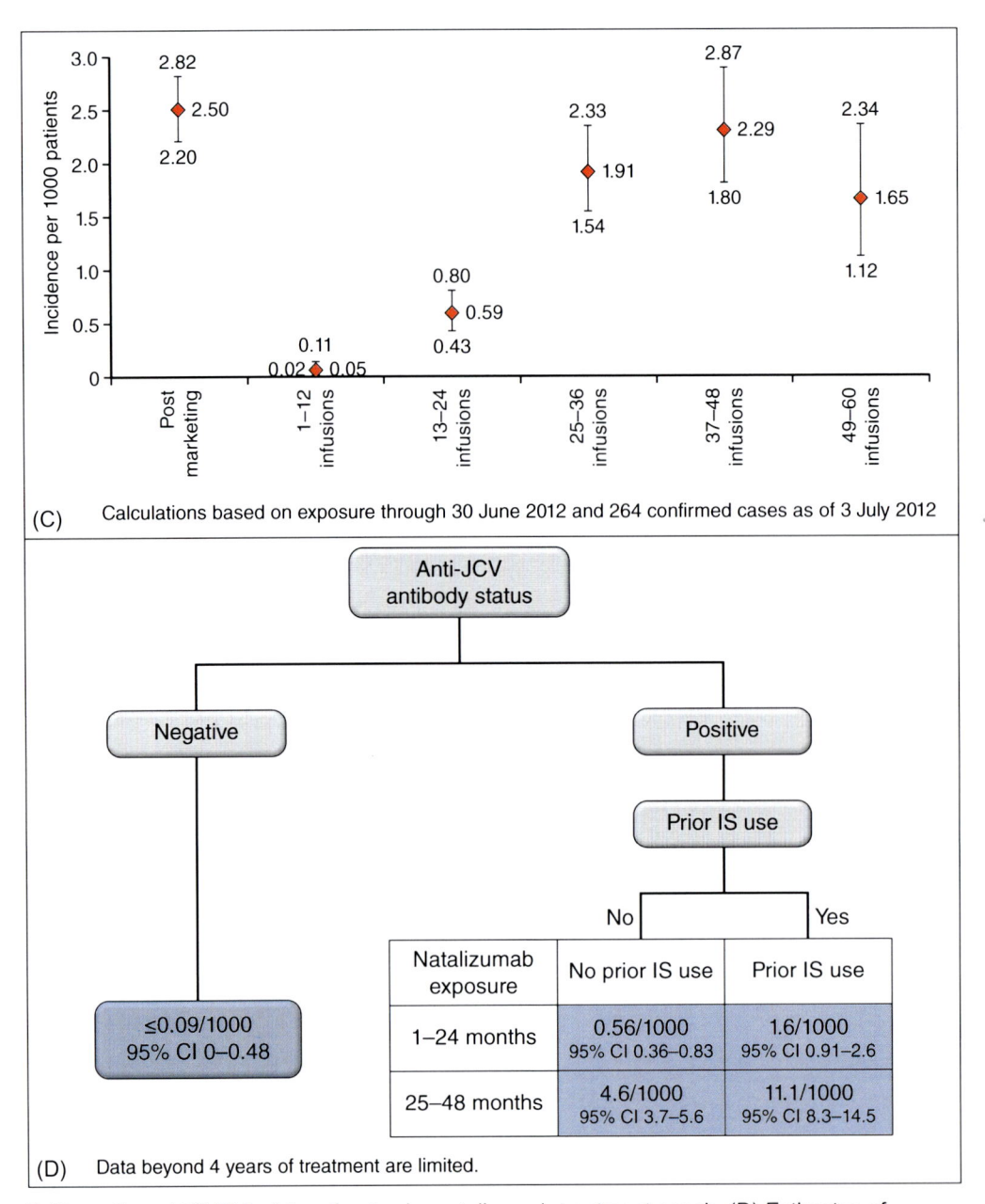

7.10 *continued* (C) PML risk estimates by natalizumab treatment epoch. (D) Estimates of PML risk in those who are JC virus seropositive and seronegative, stratified by previous immunosuppressant exposure and duration of treatment.

1. Whether the person has previously been infected with JCV; this is demonstrated by the presence of IgG directed against the capsid protein of JCV on serological testing (i.e. JCV seropositivity).
2. Previous use of immunosuppressants.
3. Duration of treatment with natalizumab. The risk increases as treatment duration increases, and is markedly increased in those who have been on treatment for >2 years.

The lowest risk of developing PML in those on natalizumab is in those who are JCV seronegative, regardless of the duration of treatment. Conversely, the highest risk is in those who have previously received immunosuppressant therapy, are JCV seropositive, and have received natalizumab for >2 years. Just under 50% of the adult MS population are JCV seronegative; the seroconversion rate in this group is approximately 0.5% per annum. It is recommended that those patients receiving natalizumab who are seronegative for JCV are tested annually to monitor for seroconversion. If they seroconvert they should then be classified as being at higher risk of developing PML.

Fingolimod (FTY720 or Gilenya®)

Fingolimod is a sphingosine-1-phosphate (S1P) receptor modulator. It binds to the S1P receptors, internalizing them and preventing them being recycled to the cell membrane. Fingolimod prevents lymphocytes from egressing out of lymph nodes, thus reducing the overall number of circulating lymphocytes. It primarily selects naïve lymphocytes. Fingolimod may also have neuroprotective actions, and may promote neuronal repair by directly modulating S1P receptor on neural and glial cells.

Fingolimod is approved as a first-line therapy in several countries. In Europe it has been approved as a second-line treatment for highly active RRMS, in those who have been shown to be non-responders to first-line DMDs. It is currently being tested in PPMS in phase III studies. Fingolimod is an oral tablet, which is taken once daily at a dose of 0.5 mg.

In clinical trials of fingolimod, the annualized relapse rate was decreased by 55–60% and a significant decrease was observed in the MRI activity parameters (new T2, Gd+ lesions and brain atrophy) compared to both placebo and IFN-β1a. Disability progression as measured by the EDSS was decreased, but only in comparison to placebo.

There are a number of side effects that were seen in the fingolimod arm of clinical trials.

1. Cardiovascular effects are relatively common and potentially serious. These are thought to be due to the presence of S1P receptors in the heart. Bradycardia has been documented in about 24% of male and about 8% of female patients; an asymptomatic bradycardia usually occurs within 6 h of the first dose and usually resolves. First-degree atrioventricular (AV) block (PR prolongation) is seen in about 1% of 20–49-year-old patients and about 8% of 50–79-year-old patients. Second-degree AV block Mobitz type I is seen (usually at night) in about 1.4% of asymptomatic healthy individuals and in individuals with resting heart rate <60 bpm. An AV block at 2:1 is rarely seen, occurring in about 0.5% of patients.
2. Additional cardiovascular risk factors, including hypertension and increased triglycerides have been documented in a minority of patients.
3. An increase in the rate of infections, including viral and respiratory tract infections, gastroenteritis and herpesvirus infections, has been associated with fingolimod.
4. Lymphopenia occurs in almost all patients on fingolimod. Additionally, patients should be monitored for the development of serological abnormalities, including increased liver enzymes (alanine aminotransferase and γ-glutamyltransferase).
5. Rarely, macular oedema has been documented in association with fingolimod, and patients at risk of this (such as those with pre-existing diabetes) must be warned about this potentially sight-threatening condition.

As a result of these potential side effects, patients receiving fingolimod must be actively monitored for the development of potentially serious complications. Monitoring requirements include the following.

1. Baseline FBC, LFT and ECG. Patients should be monitored by continuous real-time ECG for 6 h after the first dose, and an ECG should be performed yearly in all patients. If severe bradycardia persists at the end of the 6-hour monitoring period, monitoring should be extended for at least 2 h. If a patient develops symptomatic bradycardia within 24 h of the first dose they should be monitored overnight, or until symptoms resolve. If symptomatic bradycardia persists, specialist cardiological advice should be sought. First-dose monitoring should be repeated if a patient has a treatment break of 14 days or longer.
2. Ophthalmological examination should be performed in all patients to monitor for the development of macular oedema. This tends to be self-limiting and usually resolves spontaneously. Ophthalmological examination should be repeated at 3–4 months. In patients with diabetes mellitus, the ophthalmological examination should be performed regularly while the patient is on fingolimod.
3. Varicella zoster virus serology should be performed at baseline. If a patient is varicella zoster virus seronegative, they should be vaccinated against it and treatment initiation delayed for at least 6 weeks.

Mitoxantrone (Novantrone®)

Mitoxantrone is a synthetic antineoplastic anthracenedione that is able to cross the BBB and inhibit DNA replication and DNA-dependent RNA synthesis, in addition to inhibiting the ability of topoisomerase II to repair DNA. This ultimately leads to apoptosis of both proliferating and non-proliferating cells. In MS, mitoxantrone suppresses T-cell, B-cell and macrophage proliferation; decreases secretion of proinflammatory cytokines (IFN-γ, tumour necrosis factor, interleukin-2); and inhibits macrophage-mediated myelin degradation.

Mitoxantrone was approved in 2000 by the US Food and Drug Administration (FDA) for use in:

1. patients with RRMS with >2 relapses/year, with incomplete remission from relapses and an insufficient response to disease-modifying therapies;
2. patients with SPMS with marked progression of disability (>1 EDSS points/year) and/or high relapse rate;
3. patients with SPMS and PPMS with rapid progression without relapses.

The dose of mitoxantrone is 12 mg/m^2 of body surface area, which is given as a slow intravenous infusion every 3 months, up to a lifetime maximum dose of 140 mg/m^2 (about 12 infusions). An induction phase consisting of monthly infusions for the first 3 months of treatment has been suggested in highly aggressive forms of MS.

Mitoxantrone has been shown to reduce the annualized relapse rate by 66%; to reduce Gd+ and new T2 lesions by 80%; and to slow the progression of disease in patients with rapidly progressing RRMS, SPMS and PPMS.

The use of mitoxantrone is limited by safety concerns.

1. Commonly experienced side effects include nausea and vomiting (55–76%); menstrual disorders (51–61%), including persistent amenorrhoea (seen in 7% of women <35 years old and 14% of women >35 years old); urinary tract and upper respiratory tract infections; and alopecia (38–61%). Leucopenia is seen in 10–20% of patients receiving mitoxantrone.
2. Less commonly experienced, but more serious side effects limit the use of mitoxantrone in practice. These tend to be dependent on the total dose of mitoxantrone received. Compromised left ventricular ejection function (LVEF) is seen in about 12% of patients; congestive heart failure in 0.4%; and therapy-related acute leukaemia in about 0.21% of patients with long-term use. Early cardiotoxicity has been rarely reported at the time of the third dose.

Because of the potential for these serious side effects, patients receiving mitoxantrone are required to undergo monitoring both before and during treatment.

1. ECG should be performed and LVEF assessed using either echocardiogram or MUGA (radionuclide-based multiple gated acquisition scan). An assessment of LVEF should be performed at baseline and before each administration (i.e. every 3 months). These assessments should continue until 80 months after the end of treatment. If the LVEF decreases to <50%, mitoxantrone should be discontinued.
2. FBC, LFT, pregnancy test and urinalysis should be performed before each administration. If the baseline neutrophil count is <1500 cells/mm^3, or bilirubin is >3.4 mg/dl (indicating the presence of cholestasis), mitoxantrone should not be prescribed.
3. During infusions, patients should be monitored for signs of extravasation due to the risk of tissue necrosis. If extravasation occurs, the infusion should be discontinued, the arm elevated and ice packs applied. Topical corticosteroids may reduce inflammation and pain at the site of extravasation. If skin necrosis appears then surgical debridement and skin grafting may be necessary.

Treatments in the pipeline

Oral therapies

There are oral treatments that are currently close to being reviewed by the regulatory agencies and are likely to be available soon. However, regulatory approval is by no means a 'done deal'. Cladribine, a synthetic purine nucleoside that acts through depletion of lymphocytes and causes a prolonged lymphopenia, was recently reviewed. Despite its substantial efficacy (a 58% reduction in absolute risk reduction, 33% reduction in EDSS progression, 73% reduction in new T2 lesions and 86% reduction in Gd+ lesions compared to placebo) and a relatively safe profile demonstrated in the phase II and III studies versus placebo (CLARITY study)[2] and IFN-β (ORACLE study)[3], this oral medication did not achieve regulatory approval in either the EU or the USA due to concerns regarding long-term safety. Because of this, the company developing the drug decided not to pursue the global approval process. This highlights some of the problems that may be encountered when attempting to gain regulatory approval for new MS therapies, where there may be concerns regarding longer-term side effects.

BG12 (dimethyl fumarate)

BG12 exerts an immunomodulatory effect. The fumaric acid esters reduce leucocyte passage across the BBB and exert neuroprotective properties through activation of antioxidant pathways (nuclear factor E2-related factor 2 pathway). This protects against neuronal death and myelin injury related to oxidative stress.

It is an oral tablet, taken at a dose of 240 mg twice a day. The efficacy of BG12 is summarized in *Table 7.1*.

Common side effects seen in clinical trials include abdominal pain, flushing and headache. These were most marked on therapy initiation, and tended to resolve if treatment was continued for 4 weeks. Other side effects include abnormal LFT or renal function tests, lymphopenia, nasopharyngitis, nausea, and diarrhoea and vomiting. In the clinical trial setting, treatment was discontinued when abnormalities persisted for >4 weeks; however, the frequency of monitoring required in routine clinical practice remains to be determined.

Teriflunomide (Aubagio®)

Teriflunomide reduces T-cell proliferation by reducing activity of the mitochondrial enzyme dihydro-orotate dehydrogenase, which is crucial in pyrimidine synthesis. It is a 14-mg oral tablet, taken once daily. The efficacy of teriflunomide is summarized in *Table 7.1*.

Diarrhoea, nausea, abnormal LFT, paraesthesias, arthralgia and hair thinning were seen on the treatment arm of the teriflunomide trials. In addition, neutropenia, rhabdomyolysis and peripheral neuropathy may be associated with the use of teriflunomide. Teriflunomide is an active metabolite of leflunomide, which has been associated with fatal liver failure, one case of PML and possible teratogenic effects. The possible association of the risk profile of teriflunomide to that of leflunomide will be an important issue for consideration on its future use in clinical practice.

Laquinimod

The mechanism of action of laquinimod is not fully understood, but an immunomodulatory effect has been described. Laquinimod appears to inhibit T-cell and macrophage entry into the CNS. Additionally, it appears

Table 7.1 Updates on efficacy of future oral therapies

	Teriflunomide TEMSO[4] (versus placebo)	Laquinimod ALLEGRO[5] (versus placebo)	Laquinimod BRAVO[6] (versus placebo)	BG12 DEFINE[7] (versus placebo)	BG12 CONFIRM[8] (versus placebo and GA)	BAF312 BOLD[9]* (versus placebo)
Absolute risk reduction	31%	23%	21.3%	53%	44–51% versus 30% in GA	48–66%
New/enlarged T2 lesions	67%	30%	–	85%	71–73% versus 54% in GA	80%
Gd+ lesions	32–40%	37%	–	90%	65–74% versus 65% in GA	77–84%
New/enlarged T1 lesions	–	–	–	–	57–65% versus 41% in GA	–
Brain atrophy	–	33%	27.5%	–	–	–
EDSS	30%	36%	33.5%	38%	24% versus 7% in GA	–
Proportion of disease-free patients	50–52%	–	–	77%	–	77–92%

EDSS, Expanded Disability Status Score; GA, glatiramer acetate.
*BOLD study results from 6 months in the study.

to promote the anti-inflammatory profile of T cells, shifting them from a proinflammatory T-helper 1 to anti-inflammatory or regulatory T-helper 2/3 cell profile.

Laquinimod is taken as a 0.6 mg tablet once daily. There have been two phase III studies in patients with RRMS (ALLEGRO and BRAVO). The efficacy of laquinimod is summarized in *Table 7.1*.

Side effects associated with laquinimod include arthralgia, herpesvirus and urinary tract infections, gastrointestinal side effects, and abnormal LFT. Elevations of the transaminase liver enzymes were noticed, reaching three times the upper limit of normal in 5% of patients. These elevations appear to be transitory, asymptomatic and reversible.

Monoclonal antibodies

Several monoclonal antibodies have either completed, or are close to the completion of, phase II and III clinical trials and appear to show very promising results.

Alemtuzumab (Lemtrada®)

Alemtuzumab is a humanized monoclonal antibody targeting the CD52 antigen, which is present on the surface of all mature leucocytes. Alemtuzumab administration causes a rapid and profound depletion of both B and T cells. The B-cell depletion is reversed in approximately 3 months after initial treatment, with counts overshooting baseline levels, while CD4+ and CD8+ T-cell levels remain reduced for 3–9 months. Even when CD4+ and CD8+ T cells recover to above normal they rarely if ever return to pretreatment baseline levels.

Alemtuzumab is administered intravenously at a dose of 12 mg/day for 5 days in the first year and for 3 days in year 2. Third or subsequent annual courses are given thereafter based on clinical disease activity. In a phase II double-blinded study comparing alemtuzumab to IFN-β1a over 5 years, alemtuzumab lowered the risk of sustained accumulation of disability by 72% and reduced the rate of relapse by 69%. The mean disability of patients on alemtuzumab was reduced at 36 months in contrast to the IFN-β1a group, where an increase in disability was seen.

Side effects associated with alemtuzumab include headache, rash, nausea, hives, fever, pruritus, insomnia, upper respiratory and urinary tract infections, herpes infections (simplex and varicella zoster) and fatigue. Secondary autoimmunity, presumably as a result of immune system reconstitution is a well recognized complication of alemtuzumab treatment. Autoimmune thyroid disease (such as Graves' disease, **7.11**) appears to occur in about 30% of patients and idiopathic thrombocytopenic purpura in 2–3% (**7.12**). Several cases of Goodpasture's disease have also been described, along with cases of immune-mediated neutropenia and haemolytic anaemia. Patients receiving alemtuzumab therefore have to undergo regular monitoring for these conditions with investigations, including FBC, thyroid function tests, and urinary testing for Goodpasture's.

Daclizumab

Daclizumab is a humanized monoclonal antibody directed against the α-subunit of the interleukin-2 receptor (CD25), which is present on activated T cells. The mechanism of action is not well described, but it has been related to an increase in the immunoregulatory activity of CD56 natural killer cells.

Daclizumab is administered as a subcutaneous injection of 150 mg, 2 weeks apart for the first two doses and every 4 weeks thereafter.

A phase II randomized, double-blind, placebo-controlled study in 230 patients with RRMS already on IFN-β1a or IFN-β1b (the CHOICE study)[10] revealed a 72% reduction in active lesions on MRI in those patients receiving the higher dose of daclizumab (300 mg), while a phase IIb study (SELECT)[11] of daclizumab versus placebo in 600 patients with RRMS revealed a 54% reduction in absolute risk reduction in both doses (150 mg and 300 mg). An average reduction of 2.5 points on EDSS or stabilization of EDSS has been demonstrated in previous phase II studies; however due to the small sample sizes, further studies are required to establish its efficacy. A phase III (DECIDE)[12] double-blinded, placebo-controlled, comparative to intramuscular IFN-β1a study is currently ongoing.

Side effects documented in clinical trials include rash, eczema, upper respiratory tract and other infections, anaemia, paraesthesias and transient abnormal liver enzymes. Daclizumab appears to have a relatively good safety profile in comparison to other existing monoclonal antibodies, but it lacks robust data as a monotherapy in RRMS. There is great interest in ongoing studies, as it is thought that this drug shows promise as an emerging therapy in MS.

Ocrelizumab (being developed in place of rituximab)

Ocrelizumab is a humanized anti-CD20 monoclonal antibody, which depletes CD20+ B cells. It is given as an intravenous administration of 600 mg/cycle of ocrelizumab,

Treatment issues in multiple sclerosis

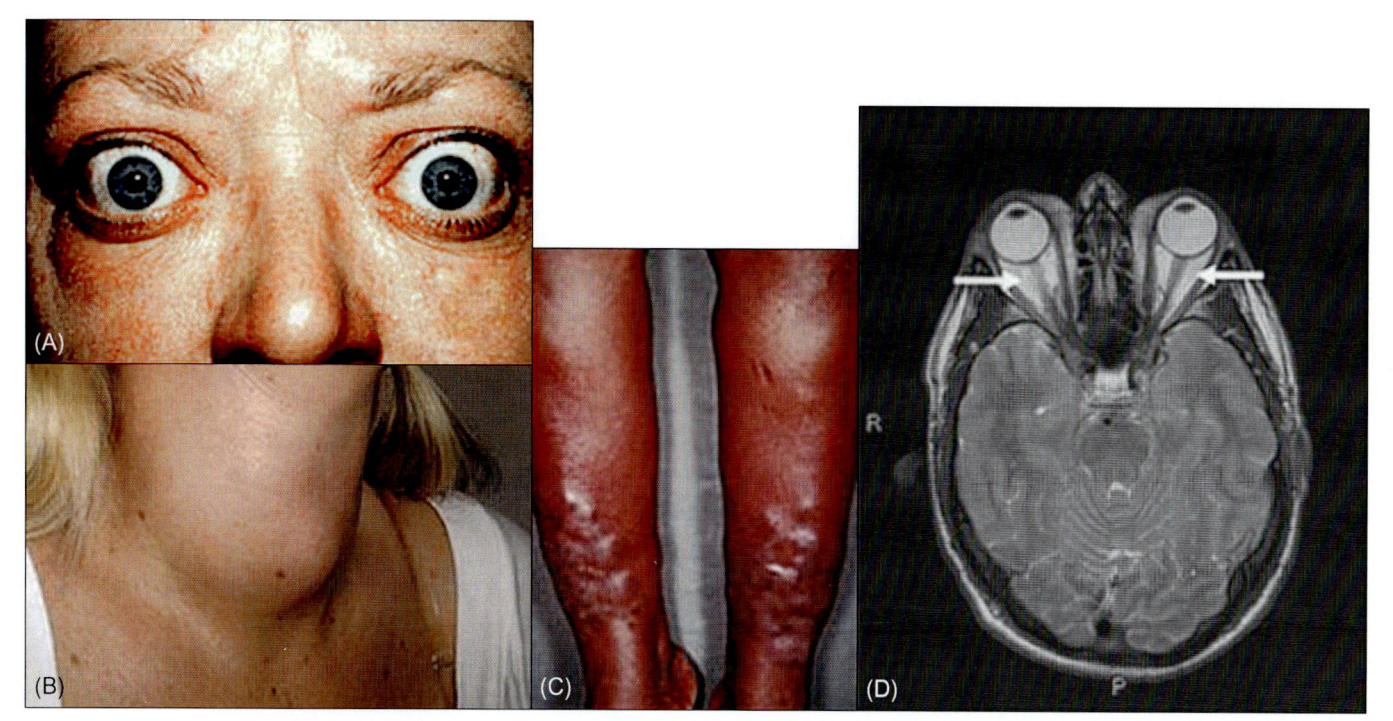

7.11 Common clinical and MRI findings in Grave's disease. (A) Grave's ophthalmopathy. (B) enlarged thyroid gland (goitre). (C) pretibial myxoedema. (D) MRI of the orbits revealing congestion of the retro-orbital space and enlargement of extraocular muscles in Grave's ophthalmopathy (*arrowed*).

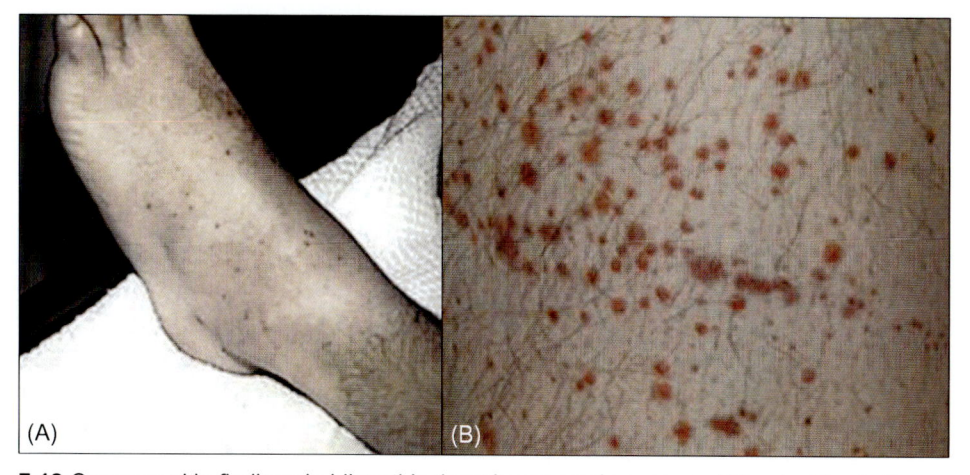

7.12 Common skin findings in idiopathic thrombocytopenic purpura. (A) petechiae in the lower limbs. (B) purpura, small bruise-like marks in association with bleeding gums or bleeding from nostrils and menorrhagia.

in two divided doses 14 days apart per cycle, for up to five to six cycles. Each cycle is repeated every 26 weeks.

A phase II, double-blind, placebo-controlled study in 218 patients with RRMS, who were randomized to ocrelizumab, IFN-β1a or placebo, revealed an 80% reduction in relapse rate and about 90% reduction of the mean number of Gd+ lesions on MRI in those patients receiving ocrelizumab compared to placebo. Ocrelizumab is currently being evaluated against IFN-β1a in two phase III studies in patients with RRMS (OPERA I and II)[13,14] and versus placebo in PPMS (ORATORIO).[15]

Relatively common side effects include infusion reactions, such as rash, pruritus and urticaria. Less commonly seen are opportunistic infections.

Conclusions

The number of drugs available for people with RRMS is increasing. This is of overall benefit to patients, but will make the choice of drugs for individual patients more challenging than when only the first-line DMDs were available. If a patient is stable and tolerating a previously prescribed treatment there should be no compelling reason to change therapy. However, patients who are not responding well to licensed DMDs, or who are JCV seropositive and have a prolonged exposure to natalizumab, should be considered for alternative second-line treatments. However, there are currently no data about the efficacy and risk profile that these patients will face after switching. For this reason decisions regarding switching to an oral agent or an investigatory agent (monoclonal antibodies) should be made on an individual basis according to both the anticipated clinical outcome and possible benefit to the patient. As we still have no way of predicting which drugs are appropriate for which individual, participation in clinical trials remains important.

Independently of the chosen drug, pretreatment investigations to identify those at higher risk of adverse side effects, and close monitoring of both clinical outcomes and adverse events during treatment are the best way to take advantage of current scientific developments.

References

1. ASCEND trial. Currently recruiting (http://clinicaltrials.gov/ct2/show/NCT01416181).
2. Giovannoni G, Comi G, Cook S, *et al*; CLARITY Study Group. A placebo-controlled trial of oral cladribine for relapsing multiple sclerosis. *N Engl J Med* 2010; **362**: 416–26.
3. ORACLE trial. Completed but results not yet published (http://clinicaltrials.gov/ct2/show/NCT00725985).
4. O'Connor P, Wolinsky JS, Confavreux C, *et al*; TEMSO Trial Group. Randomized trial of oral teriflunomide for relapsing multiple sclerosis. *N Engl J Med* 2011; **365**: 1293–303.
5. Comi G, Jeffery D, Kappos L, *et al*; ALLEGRO Study Group. Placebo-controlled trial of oral laquinimod for multiple sclerosis. *N Engl J Med* 2012; **366**: 1000–9.
6. Vollmer TL, Soelberg Sorensen P, Arnold DL, on behalf of the BRAVO Study Group. A placebo-controlled and active comparator phase III trial (BRAVO) for relapsing-remitting multiple sclerosis. Abstract and data presented at ECTRIMS 2011.
7. Gold R, Kappos L, Arnold DL, *et al*; DEFINE Study Investigators. Placebo-controlled phase 3 study of oral BG-12 for relapsing multiple sclerosis. *N Engl J Med* 2012; **367**: 1098–107.
8. Fox RJ, Miller DH, Phillips JT, *et al*; CONFIRM Study Investigators. Placebo-controlled phase 3 study of oral BG-12 or glatiramer in multiple sclerosis. *N Engl J Med* 2012; **367**: 1087–97.
9. Stuve O, Selmaj K, Li D, *et al*. BAF312, a selective sphingosine-1-phosphate receptor modulator improves MRI and clinical outcomes. Data presented at AAN 2012.
10. Wynn D, Kaufman M, Montalban X, *et al*; CHOICE investigators. Daclizumab in active relapsing multiple sclerosis (CHOICE study): a phase 2, randomised, double-blind, placebo-controlled, add-on trial with interferon beta. *Lancet Neurol* 2010; **9**: 381–90.
11. Giovannoni G, Gold R, Selmaj K, *et al*. A randomized, double-blind, placebo-controlled study to evaluate the safety and efficacy of daclizumab HYP monotherapy in relapsing-remitting multiple sclerosis: primary results of the SELECT trial. Abstract and data presented at ECTRIMS 2011.
12. DECIDE trial. Ongoing (http://clinicaltrials.gov/show/NCT01064401).
13. OPERA trial. Ongoing (http://clinicaltrials.gov/ct2/show/NCT01247324).
14. OPERA II trial. Currently recruiting (http://clinicaltrials.gov/ct2/show/NCT01412333).
15. ORATORIO trial. Currently recruiting (http://clinicaltrials.gov/ct2/show/study/NCT01194570).

Chapter 8

Clinical outcome measures in multiple sclerosis

Ruth Dobson and Ben Turner

Why do we need clinical outcome measures in multiple sclerosis?

There are an increasing number of disease-modifying drugs used in MS. To assess the efficacy of these, both in clinical trials and to ensure patients are responding to treatment, standardized sensitive and reproducible outcome measures are required.

It is unlikely that a single clinical outcome measure will be able to measure all facets of MS in even a single patient, let alone the entire patient population. Therefore, a number of outcome measures have been developed for use in MS.

Expanded Disability Status Score

The EDSS has been the gold standard for quantifying disability in MS for many years, and is used in nearly all MS clinical trials (**8.1**). EDSS assessment is carried out in person by a trained clinician. There are eight functional systems, which are each scored separately (*Table 8.1*). These scores are then combined, together with a measure of ambulation, to provide overall EDSS.

The EDSS ranges from 0 (normal neurological examination) to 10 (death due to MS) in 0.5 increments. Intermediate scores of 1.0–3.0 indicate minimal disability, 3.0–5.0 moderate disability and a score of >6.0 indicates that

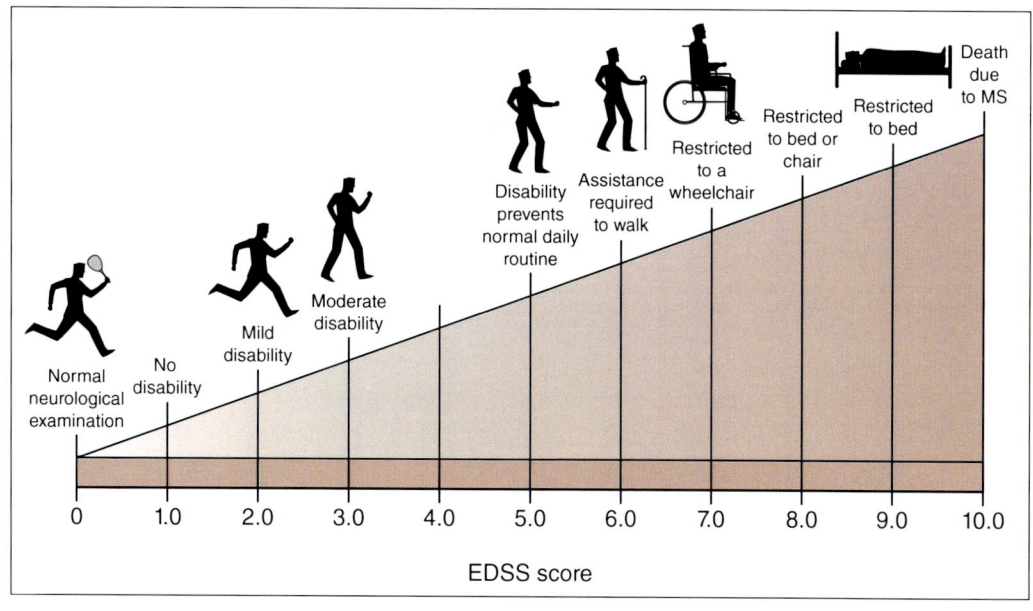

8.1 Pictorial representation of Expanded Disability Status Score.

assistance is required to walk. The EDSS has a number of advantages: it is familiar to all MS clinicians, and the entire range of disability caused by MS is encompassed within the scale.

However, the EDSS has been criticized for multiple reasons. It is a non-linear scale; an increase of 1 point on the scale at the lower end does not equate to a similar increment in disability at the upper end. The scale is heavily weighted towards walking disability and the upper end of the scale does not take into account disabilities in other areas such as upper limb and/or cognitive function. In addition, it has been argued that the EDSS is relatively insensitive to change and there are major problems with inter-rater reproducibility, especially at the lower end of the scale.[1,2]

Table 8.1 Functional systems contributing to EDSS. A score is calculated for each functional system. These are then combined with a measure of ambulation to produce the overall EDSS (see 8.1)

Functional System	Score
Vision	0 Normal
	1 Disc pallor and/or small scotoma and/or corrected acuity of worse eye <20/20
	2 Worse eye with corrected visual acuity 20/30–20/59
	3 Worse eye with large scotoma and/or moderate decrease in fields and/or corrected visual acuity 20/60–20/99
	4 Worse eye with marked decrease of fields and/or corrected visual acuity 20/100–20/200; grade 3 plus acuity of better eye <20/60
	5 Worse eye with corrected visual acuity <20/200; grade 4 plus acuity of better eye <20/60
	6 Grade 5 plus visual acuity of better eye <20/60
Brainstem	0 Normal
	1 Signs only
	2 Moderate nystagmus and/or moderate extra-ocular muscle (EOM) impairment and/or other mild disability
	3 Severe nystagmus and/or marked EOM impairment and/or moderate disability of other cranial nerves
	4 Marked dysarthria and/or other marked disability
	5 Inability to swallow or speak
Pyramidal	0 Normal
	1 Abnormal signs without disability
	2 Minimal disability, reduced performance in strenuous motor tasks
	3 Mild to moderate paraparesis or hemiparesis and/or severe monoparesis
	4 Marked paraparesis or hemiparesis or monoplegia; and/or moderate tetraparesis
	5 Paraplegia and/or marked tetraparesis and/or hemiplegia
	6 Tetraplegia
Cerebellar	0 Normal
	1 Abnormal signs without disability
	2 Mild ataxia and/or moderate Romberg sign and/or tandem walking not possible
	3 Moderate limb ataxia and/or moderate or severe gait/truncal ataxia
	4 Severe gait/truncal ataxia and severe ataxia in three or four limbs
	5 Unable to perform co-ordinated movements due to ataxia
	6 Pyramidal weakness or sensory deficits interfere with cerebellar testing

Table 8.1 *continued*

Sensory	0 Normal
	1 Mild vibration or temperature decrease in one or two limbs
	2 Mild decrease in touch, pain or position sense, or moderate decrease in vibration in one or two limbs; and/or mild vibration or temperature decrease in more than two limbs
	3 Moderate decrease in touch, pain or position sense, or marked reduction of vibration in one or two limbs; and/or mild decrease in touch or pain, or moderate decrease in all proprioceptive tests in more than two limbs
	4 Marked decrease in touch or pain in one or two limbs; and/or moderate decrease in touch or pain and/or marked reduction of proprioception in more than two limbs
	5 Loss of sensation in one or two limbs; and/or moderate decrease in touch or pain and/or marked reduction of proprioception for most of the body below the head
	6 Sensation essentially lost below the head
Bowel and bladder	0 Normal
	1 Mild urinary hesitancy, urgency and/or constipation
	2 Moderate urinary hesitancy/retention and/or moderate urinary urgency/incontinence and/or moderate bowel dysfunction
	3 Frequent urinary incontinence or intermittent self-catheterization; needs enemas or manual measures to evacuate bowels
	4 In need of almost constant catheterization
	5 Loss of bladder or bowel function; indwelling catheter
	6 Loss of bowel and bladder function
Cerebral	0 Normal
	1 Signs only in decrease in mentation; mild fatigue
	2 Mild decrease in mentation; moderate or severe fatigue
	3 Moderate decrease in mentation
	4 Marked decrease in mentation
	5 Dementia
Ambulation	0 Unrestricted
	1 Fully ambulatory (but not unrestricted)
	2 300–500 m without help or assistance (EDSS 4.5 or 5.0)
	3 200–300 m without help or assistance (EDSS 5.0)
	4 100–200 m without help or assistance (EDSS 5.5)
	5 <100 m without assistance (EDSS 6.0)
	6 >50 m with unilateral assistance (EDSS 6.0)
	7 >120 m with bilateral assistance (EDSS 6.0)
	8 <50 m with unilateral assistance (EDSS 6.5)
	9 5–120 m with bilateral assistance (EDSS 6.5)
	10 Unable to walk 5 m even with aid, uses wheelchair and transfers alone; up and about in wheelchair some 12 h/day (EDSS 7.0)
	11 Unable to take more than a few steps; may need some help in transferring and wheeling self (EDSS 7.5)
	12 Essentially restricted to bed or chair or perambulated in wheelchair, but out of bed most of day (EDSS 8.0)

Multiple Sclerosis Functional Composite

In response to the criticisms levelled at the EDSS, the Multiple Sclerosis Functional Composite (MSFC) was developed. The MSFC consists of three quantitative assessments, each examining a different modality. *z*-scores, which are a comparison between the patients' score and that of a reference population, are calculated for each section and a composite *z*-score is derived. A lower overall *z*-score represents deterioration in function.

Timed 25-foot walk
This is the time taken for the patient to walk 25 feet in ideal conditions with minimum assistance. This gives a measure of lower limb function and ambulation. Any assistance (such as the use of a walking stick) is recorded. A change of >20% in walking time is regarded as clinically significant.

Nine-hole peg test
The nine-hole peg test is a measure of arm and hand function. The task involves the patient inserting and removing nine pegs from a board (**8.2**). The time taken for this task to be performed with both the dominant and non-dominant hand is recorded, and the final score is the mean time for both hands. This is more sensitive to changes in upper limb function than the EDSS.[3]

Paced Auditory Serial Addition Test
The Paced Auditory Serial Addition Test is a measure of cognitive function. Patients listen to a series of spoken numbers separated by either a 2- or 3-second silence. Each number must be added to the previous number. The score is calculated from the proportion of correct additions.

Sloan chart (low-contrast visual acuity)

Sloan charts measure visual acuity when looking at low-contrast letters of progressively smaller size and contrast acuity (**8.3**). Sloan charts are highly sensitive to subtle visual deficits, which can be seen in MS, and they are able to detect abnormalities in a high proportion of patients with MS with 20/20 visual acuity on testing with a Snellen chart (**8.4**). They may be abnormal in people with normal VEPs, again indicating their high sensitivity for subtle visual loss.[4]

Optical coherence tomography

Optical coherence tomography is an outcome measure that is increasingly used in MS (**8.5**). It is a non-invasive method by which the retinal nerve fibre layer, which consists predominantly of unmyelinated axons, can be visualized. The change in thickness of the retinal nerve fibre layer over time provides a quantitative estimate of axonal loss. There is a

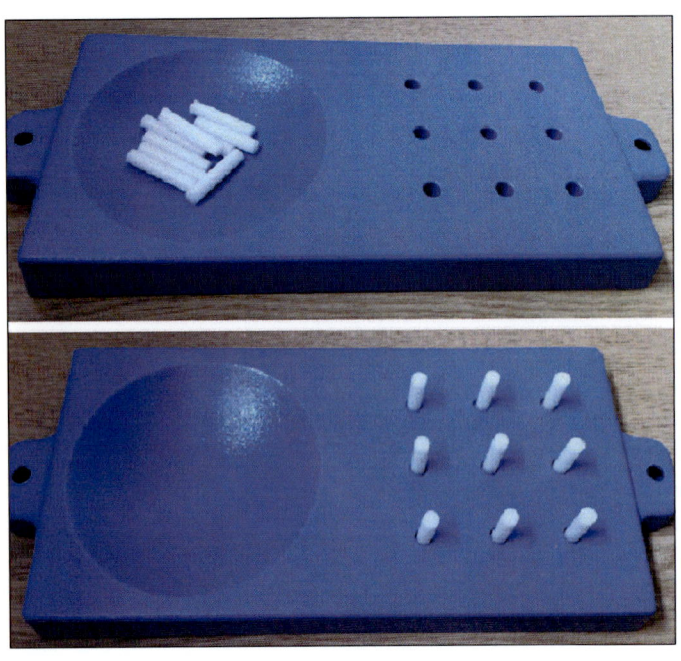

8.2 Nine-hole peg test.

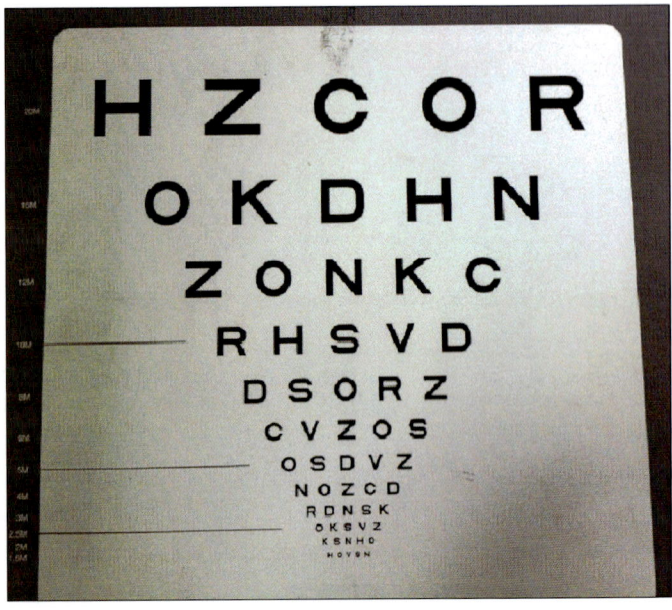

8.3 Snellen chart.

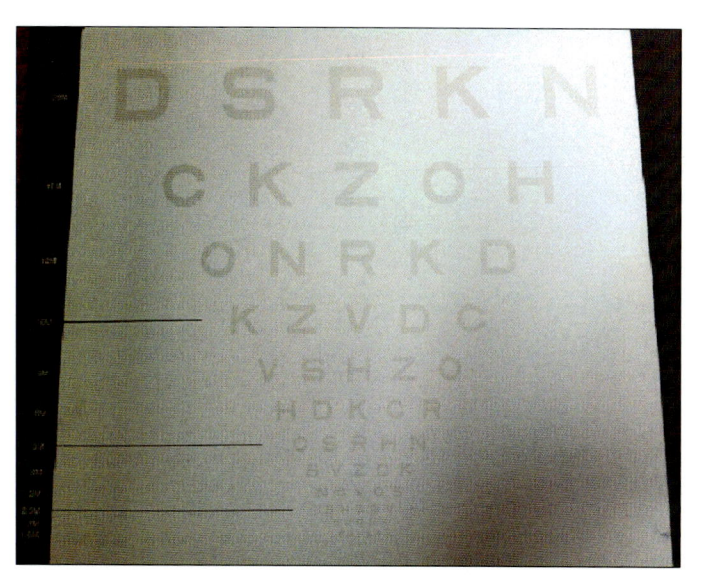

8.4 Sloan chart.

strong correlation between retinal nerve fibre layer thickness and visual acuity in those who have had optic neuritis.

The thickness of the retinal nerve fibre layer is decreased in people who have had optic neuritis within 3 months of clinical symptoms. People with MS who have not had optic neuritis also lose retinal nerve fibre layer thickness over time,[5] presumably due to axonal degeneration.

Patient-reported outcome measures

'Patient-reported outcome measure' is an umbrella term for methods used to examine the impact of MS from a patient's point of view. The tools described above all involve measurement by physicians, and they potentially miss aspects of the multifaceted ways in which MS can impact on patients' lives.

The MS Quality of Life-54 (MSQL-54) assesses the overall impact of MS on a person's quality of life by examining both generic and MS-specific impacts of disability. It is a questionnaire that patients can complete independently. This generates 12 subscales (including aspects such as physical function, social function and cognitive function) and two summary scores of physical and mental health.

The MS Impact Scale 29 (MSIS-29) was designed specifically for people with MS, and measures both the physical and psychological impact of MS. The Functional Assessment in MS (FAMS) assesses a number of symptoms, including mobility, emotional well-being, general contentment, fatigue and social well-being, and measures the level to which they affect function.

The MS walking scale is a 12-point questionnaire. It is based on the fact that walking is a complex motor activity that encompasses a number of different aspects (such as balance, co-ordination, speed, managing stairs, etc.). Patients rate the degree to which MS affects aspects of their walking ('not at all', 'a little', 'moderately', 'quite a bit' 'extremely'), and an overall score is generated.

References

1. Hobart J, Riazi A, Lamping D, Fitzpatrick R, Thompson A. Improving the evaluation of therapeutic interventions in multiple sclerosis: development of a patient-based measure of outcome. *Health Technol Assess* 2004; **8**(9): iii, 1–48.
2. Polman CH, Rudick RA. The multiple sclerosis functional composite: a clinically meaningful measure of disability. *Neurology* 2010; **74**(Suppl 3): S8–15.
3. Cutter GR, Baier ML, Rudick RA, et al. Development of a multiple sclerosis functional composite as a clinical trial outcome measure. *Brain* 1999; **122**(Pt 5): 871–82.
4. Balcer LJ, Baier ML, Cohen JA, et al. Contrast letter acuity as a visual component for the Multiple Sclerosis Functional Composite. *Neurology* 2003; **61**(10): 1367–73.
5. Petzold A, de Boer JF, Schippling S, et al. Optical coherence tomography in multiple sclerosis: a systematic review and meta-analysis. *Lancet Neurol* 2010; **9**(9): 921–32.

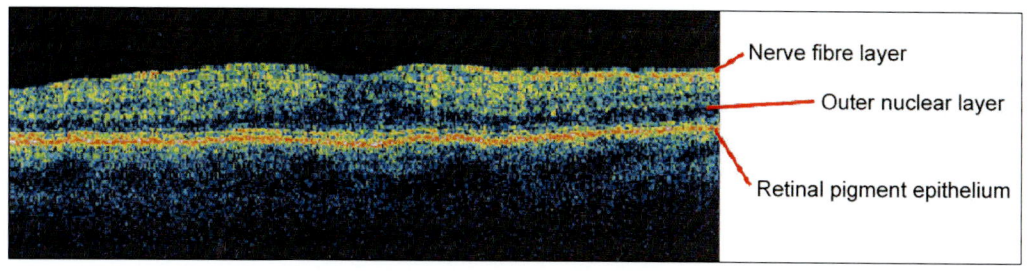

8.5 Example image obtained using optical coherence tomography.

Chapter 9

Neurorehabilitation in multiple sclerosis

Aidan Neligan, Joe Buttell and Clarence Liu

Multiple sclerosis is the most common non-traumatic cause of progressive neurological dysfunction, and rehabilitation is an important aspect in its management. As MS is a chronic condition with progression over several decades, patients have complex problems with changing needs. People with MS have multiple sites of neurological involvement, variable clinical presentations, an often unpredictable but ultimately progressive course,[1] and changing patterns of need over time. These are best managed by a multidisciplinary team, including a physician skilled in symptomatic management. Given the fluctuating nature of the condition, rehabilitation goals and the intensity of therapy can be modified over time.

What is rehabilitation?

There are various definitions of rehabilitation, all of which emphasize engaging the patient and the professionals involved in their care in both treatment and educational elements. The primary goal of rehabilitation in people with MS is to minimize functional loss and maintain functional independence despite progressive neurological impairment.[2]

In classifying patients' functions, conventionally the terms impairment, disability and handicap have been used. However, confusion may occur with the definition of the latter two terms, which have been criticized as being politically incorrect (more recently attempts have been made to substitute them with the terms activity and participation). Nevertheless, in practice they are very useful domains to use, as they allow those involved in rehabilitation to ensure that a patient's needs can be mapped out sufficiently. Other important areas include the use of appropriate outcome measures to monitor rehabilitation, and the requirement to set suitable patient-centred goals.

Rehabilitation in MS necessitates good interdisciplinary working, with complex issues best co-ordinated by an MS specialist nurse. The actual multidisciplinary rehabilitation interventions are challenging to study, although there is evidence that both inpatient and outpatient rehabilitation improves activity and participation, even without a reduction in impairment.[3,4] Nevertheless, people with MS tend to have shorter inpatient stays and make fewer improvements in activities of daily life and mobility compared to people with acute stroke or traumatic brain injury.[5]

People with MS have different rehabilitation needs throughout the disease course, as illustrated in the following case histories.

Case 1

A 35-year-old man, with a 6-year history of RRMS and previous good recovery from relapses, had mild residual bladder urgency, paroxysmal symptoms and temperature sensitivity. He was a full-time school teacher who lived with his partner and 1-year-old child in a rented property.

He had a relapse 3 months ago, treated with intravenous steroids. At the time of referral to rehabilitation services he had residual symptoms of reduced mobility, lower limb stiffness and spasms, and he had experienced falls when mobilizing. Additionally he had bladder disturbance and his sleep was poor.

On examination, he had optic atrophy, asymmetric lower limb pyramidal weakness with mild spasticity, and distal sensory disturbance. He was unable to return to work and had difficulty with childcare at home.

Case 1 is a typical scenario, with a patient with relapsing–remitting disease no longer fully recovering from relapse. In formulating rehabilitation management, it is essential to list his various difficulties, including impairments (both physical and non-physical), disabilities and handicap (activity and participation), and work through them pragmatically and holistically. In this patient, the main problems are:

1. *Weak legs.* He will benefit from neurophysiotherapy assessment and structured exercises. His spasticity may or may not require specific treatment (see below). He may require orthotics/aids (**9.1–9.5**). His visual and sensory symptoms may impact also on his gait.
2. *Bladder.* This should be investigated before commencing on medications. A toileting programme may be useful. If there is large residual volume on bladder scanning, intermittent self-catheterization may be considered.
3. *Home/work.* He may require a small care package and home adaptations to aid activities of daily life. The practicality of vocational return needs exploring.
4. *Sleep/lethargy.* It is important to distinguish between symptoms of 'MS'-associated fatigue and the impact of reactive low mood.
5. *Emotional impact* on the patient and his family should be acknowledged.

Case 2

A 49-year-old woman, with a 17-year history of MS and secondary progressive disease for the past 8 years, was walking independently with two sticks, self-transferring and able to complete upper limb tasks. She was performing intermittent self-catheterization three times a day while working part-time from home. She lives with her husband in a fully adapted house. She had a recent deterioration 1 year ago, and is now using her wheelchair more, finds it effortful to transfer, and has very clumsy hands, which affect both intermittent self-catheterization and computing.

On examination, her cognition appeared intact. She was dysarthric with ataxic upper limbs and a coarse tremor. Both legs were weak with some muscle activity on the left. There were already various adaptations made to the house/car but no input from carers. She falls when attempting to walk indoors, and uses a small self-propelling wheelchair. She has recent-onset cerebellar dysfunction with increased lower limb weakness, which has markedly increased her disability/handicap.

Case 2 is typical of someone with SPMS and highlights several issues.

1. *Dysarthria.* This leads to communication problems impacting on work. She may also need swallowing assessment via speech and language therapists.
2. *Ataxia.* Her upper limb difficulties impact on both continence care and work. She needs an occupational therapy assessment to explore management options.
3. *Weak lower limbs.* One needs to distinguish between spasticity versus 'low tone' weakness. Spasticity can be 'useful' in maintaining posture. She needs neurophysiotherapist assessment on transfer, seating and positioning with consideration of orthotics and medications (spasticity tends to be generalized).
4. *Continence.* Consider intermittent catheterization by carer/placement of suprapubic catheter and assess her toilet transfer.
5. *Social/leisure.* Her worsening has impact on her outdoor mobility, work and leisure.
6. *Care issues.* She will need an increased level of care and there may a requirement for additional adaptations, and respite for her husband should be considered.
7. *Emotional impact* on her and her family can be significant.
8. *Rehabilitation needs.* Her needs are relatively high and complex with deterioration over a short period of time. Inpatient rehabilitation may be considered.

Major symptoms and therapeutic options

The major symptoms experienced by people with MS are listed in *Table 9.1*. Particular attention needs to be paid to the 'silent symptoms', which may go unnoticed; namely fatigue, spasticity and cognitive deficits – over 40% of people with MS have cognitive deficits with the potential to affect quality of life.[6]

In the following sections, examples of symptomatic and rehabilitation therapies are discussed.

Table 9.1 Major symptoms experienced by people with MS

Fatigue	Weakness (limb, trunk, high versus low tone)
Cognitive dysfunction	Spasticity
Mood disturbances	Ataxia/gait disturbances
Visual deficits	Sensory loss
Swallowing difficulties	Pain
Speech/communication problems	Tremor
Sphincter disturbances (bladder, bowel)	Paroxysmal symptoms
Sexual dysfunction	

Gait and posture disturbances

One of the principal patient goals in MS rehabilitation is the maintenance of independence; with the importance of mobility reflected in the EDSS score (see **8.1**; *Table 8.1*).

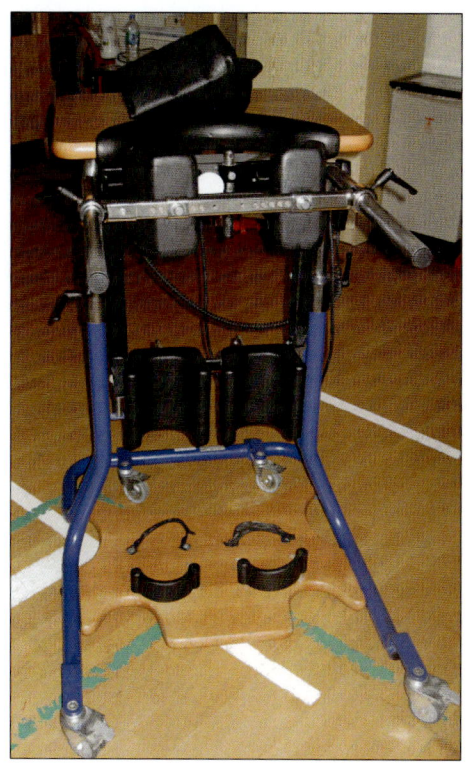

9.1 A powered standing frame provides mechanical assistance to achieve upright posture for people with leg and trunk muscle weakness, allowing them to stand.

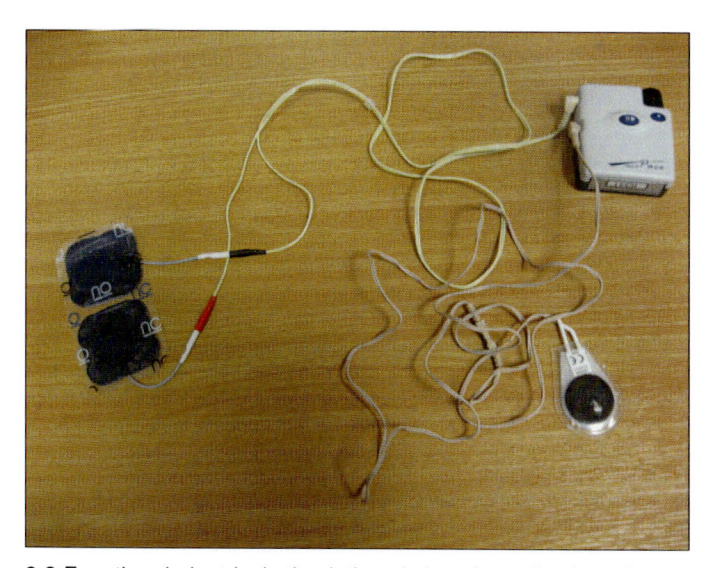

9.2 Functional electrical stimulation. A drop-foot stimulator for the management of weak anterior calf muscles: a heel switch activates the muscle stimulator at the right time to lift the weak foot when walking.

Spasticity

Spasticity refers to the velocity-dependent resistance to muscle stretch, and in practice must be distinguished from upper motor neuron syndrome or else many patients become 'over-treated'.

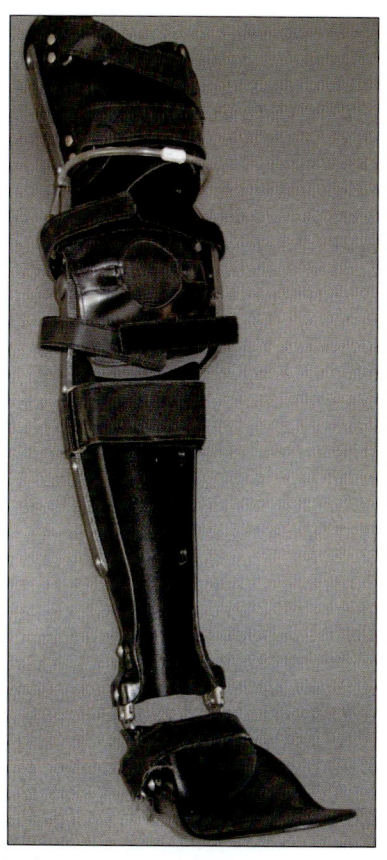

9.3 Knee–ankle–foot orthosis used for the long-term management of knee/ankle/foot weakness.

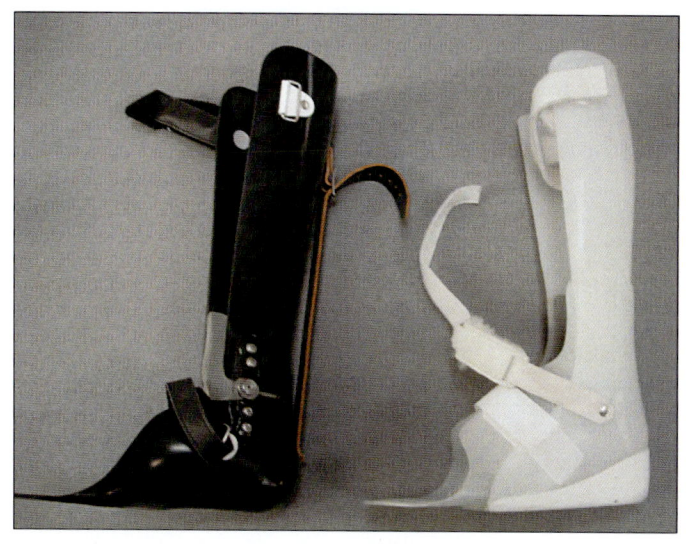

9.4 Resting splints used for the maintenance of ankle range of motion in people unable to stand or walk.

This can be managed by a combination of corrected posture, physiotherapy, oral medication (benzodiazepine, baclofen, and tinzanidine) and intrathecal baclofen pump placement for generalized spasticity (9.6). Phenol injections can be considered for intractable cases. Botulinum injections are occasionally used in people with focal spasticity.

In summary, rehabilitation goals in MS are a changing target because of the progressive nature of the condition, with the aim of maintaining functional independence and prevention of potential complications (e.g. gait training, bladder/bowel management, use of adaptive equipment) in people with neurological dysfunction.

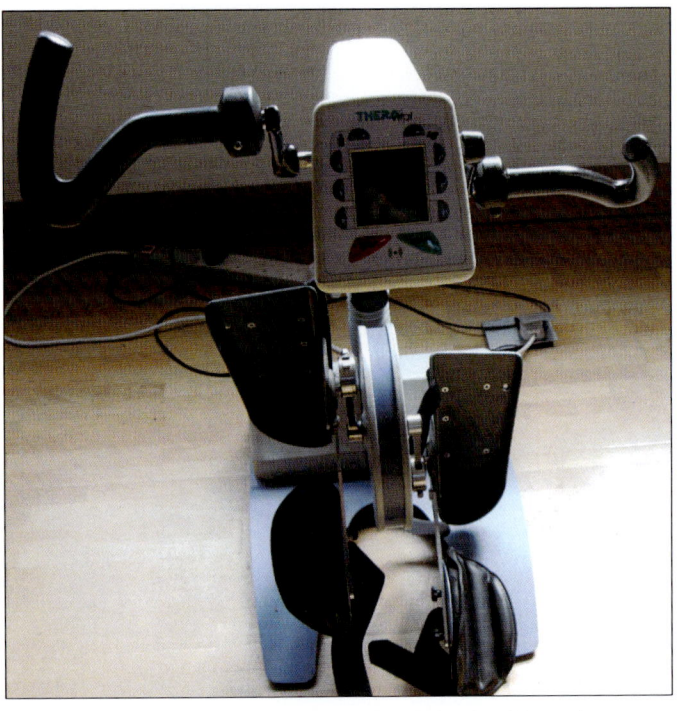

9.5 Assisted seated exercise bike allows those without the balance required to use a typical seated bike to exercise. The pedals and handles both move and assist individuals with weakness to move through the whole motion.

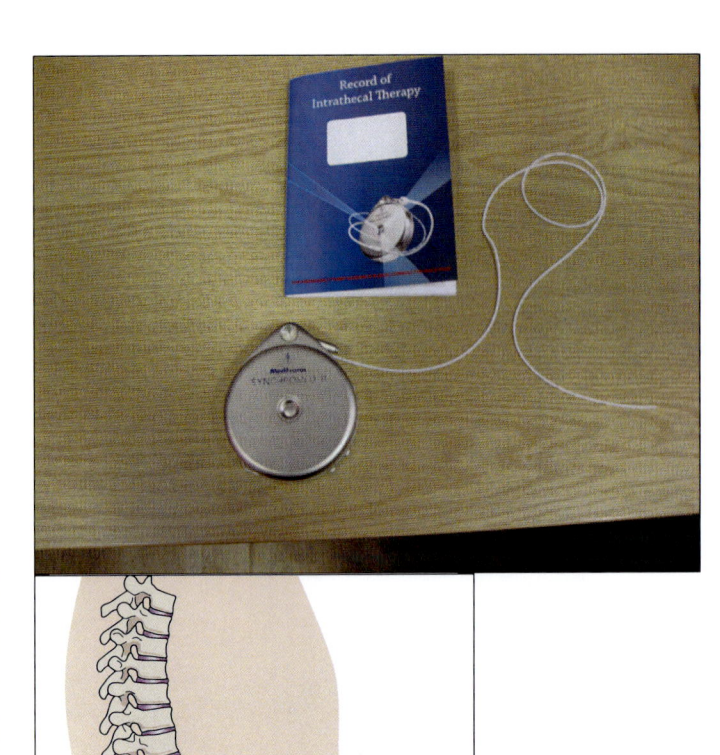

9.6 An intrathecal baclofen pump with a spinal catheter is used for the management of generalized spasticity.

References

1. Pittock SJ, Mayr WT, McClelland RL, *et al.* Change in MS-related disability in a population-based cohort: a 10-year follow-up study. *Neurology* 2004; **62**: 51–9.
2. Stevenson VL, Playford ED. Rehabilitation and MS. *Int MS J* 2007; **14**: 85–92.
3. Khan F, Turner-Strokes L, Ng L, Kilpatrick TJ. Multidisciplinary rehabilitation for adults with multiple sclerosis. *Cochrane Database Syst Rev* 2007; **2**: CD006036.
4. Khan F, Pallant JF, Brand C, Kilpatrick TJ. Effectiveness of rehabilitation intervention in persons with multiple sclerosis: a randomised controlled trial. *J Neurol Neurosurg Psychiatry* 2008; **79**: 1230–5.
5. Carey RG, Seibert JH, Posavac EJ. Who makes the most progress in inpatient rehabilitation? An analysis of functional gain. *Arch Phys Med Rehabil* 1988; **69**: 337–43.
6. Rao SM, Leo GI, Bernardin L, Unverzagt F. Cognitive dysfunction in multiple sclerosis 1. Frequency, patterns and prediction. *Neurology* 1991; **41**: 685–91.

INDEX

Note: page numbers in *italics* refer to figures and tables.

ABH mouse, EAE 45–6
active lesions 40, *41*
  MRI 21
acute disseminated encephalomyelitis (ADEM) 34
  MRI *35*
age at diagnosis 1, *2*
alemtuzumab 62
ALLEGRO study *61*, 62
allergic reactions
  to glatiramer acetate 55
  to natalizumab 56
amantadine 51
ambulation
  EDSS scores *67*
  MS walking scale 69
anaphylaxis
  after glatiramer acetate 55
  after natalizumab 56
animal models 44
  impact of studies on human treatments 48
  see also experimental autoimmune encephalomyelitis (EAE)
ASCEND trial, natalizumab 56
assisted seated exercise bikes 74
astrocytes 24
ataxia 5
  rehabilitation 72
atraumatic needles, lumbar puncture 6
atrioventricular block, after fingolimod 59
Aubagio® (teriflunomide) 61
autoimmunity 44
  complications of alemtuzumab 62, *63*
Avonex® 54
  see also interferon (IFN)-β

baclofen 51, 74
'benign MS' 3
Betaferon® 52–3
  see also interferon (IFN)-β
BG12 60–1
'black hole' lesions 21
  MRI *19*, 20
bladder distension, ultrasound scan, EAE *50*
bladder dysfunction
  EDSS scores *67*
  rehabilitation 72
blood tests 37
blood–brain barrier
  abnormalities 43
  in EAE 45
BOLD study 61
botulinum injections 74
bowel function, EDSS scores *67*
bradycardia, after fingolimod 59
brain atrophy 20, 21
brain biopsy 36
brainstem, acute infarction, MRI *33*
brainstem auditory evoked potentials (BAEPs) 28–9
brainstem functional system, EDSS scores *66*
brainstem syndromes 5
BRAVO study *61*, 62

C57BL/6 mouse
  EAE 45
  optic neuritis *47*
carbamazepine 51
cardiovascular side effects
  fingolimod 59
  mitoxantrone 60
care issues 72
central axons
  demyelination 24
  differences from peripheral axons 23–4
central motor conduction time (CMCT) 27
cerebellar functional system, EDSS scores *66*
cerebral functional system, EDSS scores *67*
cerebrospinal fluid (CSF) analysis 5–6, 36–7
cerebrovascular disease
  acute brainstem infarction *33*
  acute middle cerebral artery stroke *33*
  mimicking of MS *36*, *37*
cervical disc prolapse *35*, *38*
Charcot, Jean-Martin *39*
childhood onset MS, sex ratio 9
CHOICE study 62
chronic active lesions 40, *41*
chronic inactive lesions 40, *42*
cladribine 60

CLARITY study 60
clinical courses of MS *1*, 3
clinical outcome measures 65
  Expanded Disability Status Score 65–6
  Multiple Sclerosis Functional Composite 68
  optical coherence tomography 68–9
  patient-reported measures 69
  Sloan chart 68, *69*
clinical presentation 1, 3
  brainstem syndromes 5
  McDonald diagnostic criteria *2*
  optic neuritis 3
  presenting symptoms *2*
  'red flags' *2*
  transverse myelitis 3–4
clinical trials, use of MRI 20–1
clinically isolated syndrome 3
  first-line DMDs 52
combined unique active lesions 21
CONFIRM study 61
continuous conduction 23, *24*
convulsions, after glatiramer acetate 55
Copaxone® 54–5
  see also glatiramer acetate
cranial nerve palsies 5
cutting needles, lumbar puncture 5–6
CYP27B1 11

DA rat, EAE 46
daclizumab 62
DEFINE study 61
demyelination
  in animal models *46*
  central axons 24
  continuous conduction *24*
  MRI *7*
  physiological effects 23
demyelination models 44
depression 52
Devic's disease (neuromyelitis optica) 4, *32*
diabetes mellitus, and fingolimod 59
diagnosis 31
  McDonald criteria *2*, 19
  MRI 18–19
  'red flags' *2*

diagnosis – *continued*
    see also clinical presentation;
        differential diagnosis;
        investigations
differential diagnosis
    erroneous diagnosis of MS *38*
    primary progressive MS *34*
    relapses *32–4*
    secondary progressive MS *34, 35*
    specific MS mimics *36*
dimethyl fumarate (BG12) *60–1*
disease-modifying drugs
        (DMDs) *51*
    first-line *52–5*
    second-line *56–60*
dysarthria, rehabilitation *72*
dyspnoea, after glatiramer acetate *54*

environmental factors
    effect sizes *12*
    Epstein–Barr virus *12, 13*
    smoking *13, 14*
    vitamin D deficiency *12*
epidemiology
    environmental factors *12–13*
    genetic associations *10–11*
    global distribution *9*
    migration studies *9–10*
    month of birth effect *10*
    sex ratio *9, 10*
Epstein–Barr virus *12, 13*
evoked potential tests *24, 37*
    brainstem auditory evoked
            potentials *28–9*
    motor evoked potentials *27, 28*
    somatosensory evoked
            potentials *26–7, 28*
    visual evoked potentials *25, 25–6*
exercise bikes *74*
Expanded Disability Status Score
        (EDSS) *65–6*
    scoring system *66–7*
experimental autoimmune
        encephalomyelitis (EAE)
    bladder distension, ultrasound
            scan *50*
    evaluation of studies *46*
    impact of studies on human
            treatments *48*
    induction *44*
    neurological course *45–6, 48*
    pathology *44–5, 46*
        glial response *50*
        perivascular lesion *46*
Extavia® *52–3*
    see also interferon (IFN)-β

external ophthalmoplegia *5*
extravasation management,
        mitoxantrone *60*

familial recurrence risk *10*
fatigue *72*
    symptomatic therapies *51*
fingolimod *59*
    restriction of use *51*
first-line disease-modifying
        drugs *51, 52*
    glatiramer acetate *54–5*
    interferon (IFN)-β *52–4*
flexor spasms *4*
flu-like symptoms, after IFN-β *52*
flushing, after glatiramer acetate *54*
focal dystonia *5*
FTY720 (fingolimod) *59*
    restriction of use *51*
Functional Assessment in MS
        (FAMS) *69*
functional electrical stimulation *73*

gabapentin *51*
gait and posture disturbances,
        rehabilitation *73*
genetic associations *10–11*
Gilenya® (fingolimod) *59*
    restriction of use *51*
glatiramer acetate (GA) *52, 54–5*
glial response, EAE *50*
global distribution of MS *9*
goitre *63*
Goodpasture's disease *62*
Graves' disease *62, 63*
grey matter lesions *42–3*
gross pathology *39*

HAL-DRB1 alleles *11*
hereditary spastic paraparesis *34*
herpes zoster *56*
histology *22*
    demyelination, EAE *46*
    glial response, EAE *50*
    grey matter lesions *42–3*
    perivascular lesion, EAE *46*
    white matter lesions *39–42*
human leukocyte antigen (HLA)
        associations *10–11*

idiopathic thrombocytopenic
        purpura *62, 63*
IgG, oligoclonal bands *6*
immunosuppression
    impact on animal models of
            MS *46, 48*

induction therapy *51*
    limitations *48*
inactive lesions *40, 42*
induction therapy *51*
infection risk
    fingolimod *59*
    mitoxantrone *60*
    natalizumab *57*
infectious mononucleosis *12, 13*
information sources, online
        resources *8*
infratentorial lesions, MRI *18*
infusion-related reactions *51*
    natalizumab *56, 57*
    ocrelizumab *63*
injection-site reactions
    glatiramer acetate *55*
    IFN-β *52*
'inside-out' hypothesis *44*
interferon (IFN)-β *52*
    interferon-β1a *54*
    interferon-β1b *52–3*
internuclear ophthalmoplegia *5*
intracortical lesions *42*
intrathecal baclofen pumps *74*
investigations *36–7*
    blood tests *5*
    CSF analysis *5–6*
    magnetic resonance imaging *7*
    neurophysiology *7*
    see also magnetic resonance
            imaging
ion channel redistribution, role
        in progressive neurological
        deficit *49*

JC virus reactivation, PML *57–9*
juxtacortical lesions, MRI *18*

knee–ankle–foot orthosis *73*

laquinimod *61–2*
leg weakness, rehabilitation *72*
Lemtrada® (alemtuzumab) *62*
leucocorticoid lesions *42*
leucopenia, after mitoxantrone *60*
Lewis rat, EAE *46*
Lhermitte's syndrome *3*
lipoatrophy *55*
liver dysfunction
    after fingolimod *59*
    after IFN-β *52*
    after natalizumab *56*
local circuit current flow *23*
longitudinally extensive transverse
        myelitis *4*

Index

lumbar puncture 5–6
lupus 34
lymph node enlargement 55
lymphocytes, role in EAE 44, 45
lymphopenia
    after fingolimod 59
    after IFN-β 52

macular oedema 59
magnetic resonance imaging (MRI) 7, 17, 36
    acute brainstem infarction 33
    acute disseminated encephalomyelitis 35
    acute left middle cerebral artery stroke 33
    cervical disc prolapse 35, 38
    in clinical trials 20–1
    diagnostic use 18–19
    future developments 21
    indices 21
    neuromyelitis optica (Devic's disease) 32
    physics 17–18
    post mortem brain scanning 22
    prognostic use 20
    progressive multifocal leukoencephalopathy 56
    sarcoid lesion, cervical spine 34
    transverse myelitis 4
McDonald diagnostic criteria 2, 19
medically unexplained symptoms (MUS) 36
menstrual disorders, after mitoxantrone 60
methylprednisolone
    in optic neuritis 3
    in relapses 51
middle cerebral artery stroke, MRI 33
migraine aura 32, 36
mitoxantrone 59–60
modafinil 51
models of demyelination 44
    see also experimental autoimmune encephalomyelitis (EAE)
monitoring requirements
    alemtuzumab 62
    fingolimod 59
    mitoxantrone 60
monoclonal antibodies
    alemtuzumab 62
    daclizumab 62
    natalizumab 56–9
    ocrelizumab 62–3
monoclonal gammopathies 52

month of birth effect 10, 12
motor evoked potentials 27, 28
MS Impact Scale 29 (MSIS-29) 69
MS Quality of Life-54 (MSQL-54) 69
MS walking scale 69
Multiple Sclerosis Functional Composite (MSFC) 68
myelin, physiology 23
myelograms 34

natalizumab 56–9
    restriction of use 51
nausea and vomiting, after mitoxantrone 60
neuromyelitis optica (Devic's disease) 4, 32
neurophysiology 7
neuroprotective agents 51
    impact on animal models of MS 46, 48
neurorehabilitation 71
    case studies
        relapsing-remitting MS 71–2
        secondary progressive MS 72
        gait and posture disturbances 73
        spasticity 73–4
neutralizing antibodies (NAbs)
    in IFN-β therapy 52
    in natalizumab therapy 57
nine-hole peg test 68
normal-appearing white matter 39, 40
Novantrone® (mitoxantrone) 59–60
nystagmus 5

ocrelizumab 62–3
Oil-red-O-positive material 40, 41
oligoclonal IgG bands 6, 36–7
oligodendrocytes 23–4
    in active lesions 40
online resources 8
OPERA studies 63
optic atrophy 3, 4
optic disc, normal appearance 3
optic neuritis 3
    animal model 47
    differential diagnosis 32
    MRI 4
    papillitis 4
    visual evoked potentials 25
optical coherence tomography 68–9
ORACLE study 60
oral therapies
    fingolimod 59
    treatments in the pipeline 60–2

ORATORIO study 63
'outside-in' hypothesis 44

paced auditory serial addition test 68
pain control 51
palpitations, after glatiramer acetate 54
papillitis 3, 4
parent-of-origin effects 10, 11
pathology
    EAE 44–5, 46
    grey matter lesions 42–3
    gross lesions 39
    vascular damage 43
    white matter lesions 39–42
patient-reported outcome measures 69
periventricular lesions, MRI 18
phenol injections 74
post mortem brain scanning 22
preactive lesions 40
precession 17
pregabalin 51
presenting symptoms 3
    frequencies 2
pretibial myxoedema 63
primary progressive MS (PPMS) 3
    clinical course 1
    diagnosis 31
    differential diagnosis 34
    fingolimod 59
    mitoxantrone 60
    ocrelizumab 63
    sex ratio 9
prognosis, role of MRI 20
progressive multifocal leukoencephalopathy (PML) 57–9
    hypothetical risk stratification 57–8
    MRI 56
progressive neurological deficit, possible mechanism 49
progressive relapsing MS 3
pseudoatrophy 21
pseudolymphoma 55
pseudo-relapse 32
pupillary defects 3
pyramidal functional system, EDSS scores 66
pyrexia, pseudo-relapse 32

questionnaires, clinical outcome measures 69
Quincke needles 5–6

Ranvier, nodes of 23
Rebif® 54, *55*
   see also interferon (IFN)-β
'red flags' 2
rehabilitation 71
   case studies
      relapsing-remitting MS 71–2
      secondary progressive MS 72
   gait and posture disturbances 73
   spasticity 73–4
relapses
   definition 3
   diagnosis 31
   differential diagnosis 32–4
   treatment 51
relapsing-remitting MS (RRMS) 3
   clinical course *1*
   daclizumab 62
   fingolimod 59
   first-line DMDs 52
   mitoxantrone 60
   MRI lesions *19, 20*
   natalizumab 56
   ocrelizumab 63
   rehabilitation 71–2
   sex ratio 9
relaxation curves, MRI *18*
remyelination 24, 42
   animal models 48
renal dysfunction, cautions with glatiramer acetate 55
resting splints 73
retinal nerve fibre layer thickness
   optical coherence tomography 68–9
   reduction in optic neuritis 47

sarcoidosis, cervical spine lesion, MRI *34*
scar lesions 39
Schwann cells 24
seasonality, month of birth effect 10
second-line disease-modifying drugs 51
   fingolimod 59
   mitoxantrone 59–60
   natalizumab 56–9
secondary progressive MS (SPMS) 3
   clinical course *1*
   diagnosis 31
   differential diagnosis 34, *35*

first-line DMDs 52
mitoxantrone 60
natalizumab 56
rehabilitation 72
SELECT study 62
sensory functional system, EDSS scores 67
sex ratio 9, *10*
shadow plaques 24, 42
shingles 56
side effects of treatments
   alemtuzumab 62
   BG12 61
   daclizumab 62
   fingolimod 59
   glatiramer acetate 54–5
   interferon (IFN)-β 52
   laquinimod 62
   mitoxantrone 60
   natalizumab 56–9
   ocrelizumab 63
   teriflunomide 61
sixth nerve palsies 5
SJL mouse, EAE 45–6
Sloan chart 68, *69*
smoking 13, *14*
sodium channels 23
   redistribution, role in progressive neurological deficit *49*
somatization 36
somatosensory evoked potentials (SSEPs) 26–7, *28*
spasticity
   rehabilitation 73–4
   symptomatic therapies 51
spinal MRI *18*, 36
Sprotte needle systems 6
standing frames 73
steroids
   in optic neuritis 3
   in relapses 51
stroke, middle cerebral artery, MRI *33*
subpial lesions 42
subtypes of MS *1*
suicidal ideation 52
sunlight intensity, relationship to MS prevalence *13*
symptomatic therapies 51
   animal models 48
symptoms 72
systemic capillary leak syndrome 52

T1 relaxation, MRI 17, *18*
T2 lesions 21
T2 relaxation, MRI *18*
tachycardia, after glatiramer acetate 54
TEMSO study *61*
teriflunomide 61
third nerve palsy 5
thyroid disease, autoimmune 62, *63*
timed 25-foot walk 68
tizanidine 51
torticollis 5
transcranial magnetic stimulation 27, *27–8*
transverse myelitis 3–4
   MRI *4*
traumatic needles, lumbar puncture 5–6
treatment
   conclusions 64
   first-line disease-modifying drugs 52–5
   second-line disease-modifying drugs 56–60
treatment strategies 51
treatment types 51
treatments in the pipeline
   monoclonal antibodies 62–3
   oral therapies 60–2
trigeminal neuralgia 5
tropical spastic paraparesis 34
Tysabri® (natalizumab) 56–9
   restriction of use 51

Uhthoff's phenomenon 23

vascular damage 43
vasodilation, after glatiramer acetate 54
vision
   EDSS scores 66
   Sloan chart 68
visual evoked potentials (VEPs) 25, *25–6*, 37
   erroneous diagnosis of MS *38*
vitamin D deficiency 11, *12*

websites *8*
white matter lesions 39–42

z-score, MSFC 68